Health Care Cost Management

HEALTH CARE COST MANAGEMENT

Private Sector Initiatives

PETER D. FOX
WILLIS B. GOLDBECK
JACOB J. SPIES

HEALTH ADMINISTRATION PRESS
Ann Arbor, Michigan
1984

Library of Congress Cataloging in Publication Data

Fox, Peter D.
  Health care cost management.

  Bibliography: p.
  Includes index.
  1. Medical care—Cost control. 2. Medical economics—
United States. I. Goldbeck, Willis B., 1943–   .
II. Spies, Jacob J. III. Title: [DNLM: 1. Cost Control.
2. Economics, Hospital—United States. 3. Economics,
Medical—United States. 4. Hospital Administration—
economics—United States. WX 157 H4338]
  RA413.5.U5F68   1984   362.1′042   84–12993
  ISBN 0–910701–00–8

Health Administration Press
The University of Michigan
1021 East Huron
Ann Arbor, Michigan 48109
(313) 764-1380

Contents

Contributors

JOHN FRIEDLAND is director of technical assistance at Boston University's Center for Industry and Health Care. He has worked with physician, hospital, insurance, government, consumer, and business organizations on a variety of cost-containment activities. Projects have ranged from the preparation of consumer guidebooks for CHAMPUS and Medicare beneficiaries to the development and assessment of health maintenance organizations. He received his M.A. degree in regional planning and an A.B. degree from Cornell University. He has authored or coauthored a number of articles appearing in professional journals as well as books on health maintenance organizations, corporate "right to know" obligations, and planning and evaluating in-house corporate medical department activities.

ANNE K. KIEFHABER has worked in numerous capacities for the Washington Business Group on Health where she is now the director of the Institute on Worksite Wellness. She has been the business representative on health issues to the President's Commission on Private Sector Initiatives, conducted projects with the American Cancer Society, represented the WBGH in development of the U.S. Department of Health and Human Services' Objectives for the Nation (in health promotion and disease prevention), and directed numerous consulting projects with major employers and health policy groups. In 1984, Ms. Kiefhaber was appointed as the coordinator of worksite wellness for the U.S. Department of Health and Human Services. Ms. Kiefhaber has a B.S. in nursing from Duke University.

EILEEN J. TELL is senior research associate at Boston University's Center for Industry and Health Care. She has analyzed health cost-containment activities of industry, including those relating to HMOs, PPOs, benefit design, and coalitions. She has also recently completed a two-year study of educational, organizational, financial, and other strategies to change physicians' behavior toward more cost-effective care. She has an M.P.H. degree from the University of Michigan and a B.S. degree from Tufts University. She has written articles on a variety of topics including physicians' behavior, private sector cost-containment initiatives, end-stage renal disease, mental health, HMOs, ambulatory care, and population planning.

DIANA CHAPMAN WALSH is director of program evaluation and publications at Boston University's Center for Industry and Health Care and associate professor of social and behavioral sciences and health services in the School of Public Health. She is also coeditor of the ongoing Industry and Health Care Series, nine volumes of which were published by Springer-Verlag, the tenth by Ballinger Publishing Company. She recently completed a study, entitled "Medicine as Management: The Corporate Medical Director's Complex and Changing Role," which draws on the experience of 29 major American corporations. Dr. Walsh is currently principal investigator of a randomized controlled trial of alternative treatments for problem drinkers identified on the job, which is being conducted at General Electric Company. Dr. Walsh has published widely on subjects related to the organization, financing, and delivery of health services. She has an A.B. from Wellesley College and a master's in journalism and a Ph.D. in health policy from Boston University.

ANDREW WEBBER is the excutive vice-president of the American Medical Peer Review Association, the national trade association for PSROs and PROs. During the time this book was being written, he served as vice-president of the Washington Business Group on Health. In that capacity, he managed the organization's legislative and regulatory information services and directed the various WBGH activities that focused on utilization review. Prior to working with the WBGH, Mr. Webber was the vice-president of Public Policy Communications, Inc., where he conducted projects on citizen participation and urban policy, and provided staff assistance for the White House Conference on Balanced National Growth and Economic Development. Mr. Webber has an A.B. from Harvard College.

Preface

The early 1980s have witnessed accelerated changes in the health care delivery system and intensified public and private efforts to restrain the rise in medical costs. For example, employers, for whom expenditures for health benefits typically exceed 7 percent of pay, are beginning to take forceful actions to manage health care costs. The magnitude of these actions could not have been foreseen even a few years ago. Also, largely in response to budget pressures, federal and state governments have introduced reforms that are having major effects on the delivery system. Most notable among these reforms are the adoption of prospective payment systems for hospital services, replacing a system that reimburses hospitals for whatever their costs happen to be, and measures to promote enrollment in prepaid health plans.

Competition among providers of health care is increasing. Many hospitals are entering new markets, such as wellness programs, new ambulatory care programs, long-term care, and housing for the elderly, to generate both revenues and patient referrals. Some fee-for-service medical groups are conducting market research and are actively marketing for the first time.

This book constitutes an overview of private sector initiatives directed toward health care cost containment from the perspective of private purchasers of group coverage, mostly employers and unions. Its purpose is to synthesize what is known about various types of private sector initiatives: plan design, alternative delivery systems (health maintenance organizations and preferred provider organizations), private utilization review, health care coalitions, worksite wellness programs, new activities of corporate medical departments, and cost-containment activities of hospital trustees. It describes cost-management efforts that warrant further attention and specific initiatives that may serve as models for those engaged in cost-containment activities.

This book is adapted from work performed as part of a project to analyze private sector cost-containment initiatives funded by the Office of the Assistant Secretary for Planning and Evaluation in the U.S. Department of Health and Human Services. That project was a joint venture of Lewin and Associates, Inc., the Center for Industry and Health Care at Boston University, and the Washington Business Group on Health. Peter D. Fox of Lewin and Associates served as project director and overall editor, Jacob J. Spies served as the leader from Boston University, and Willis B. Goldbeck served as the leader from the Washington Business Group on Health. Individual chapters were also authored or coauthored by Anne K. Kiefhaber and Andrew Webber of the Washington Business Group on Health and by Diana Chapman Walsh, John Friedland, and Eileen J. Tell from Boston University.

The authors have benefited greatly from the able guidance of Marilyn Falik, who served as the federal project officer. We are also grateful for the comments and suggestions of other staff in the Office of the Assistant Secretary for Planning and Evaluation. In addition, the following consultants assisted in a variety of ways: Walter McClure, President, Center for Policy Studies; Ruth Stack, Executive Director, National Association of Employers on Health Care Alternatives; and Harry L. Sutton, Jr., Vice-President of Towers, Perrin, Forster, and Crosby (all, coincidentally, from Minneapolis). Finally, we deeply appreciate the help of the many individuals who are at the forefront of the development and administration of the initiatives described. Without them, this book could not have been written.

Examples are cited throughout of actions or programs of specific purchasers, third-party payers, providers, and other organizations. Of necessity, these examples do not constitute an exhaustive compendium, in part because the rate of innovation and change is so rapid. Thus, we apologize to those responsible for the many initiatives whose accomplishments are not mentioned.

Needless to say, any views reflected herein are those of the authors alone and, in particular, do not necessarily reflect the positions or policies of the U.S. Department of Health and Human Services.

PETER D. FOX
WILLIS B. GOLDBECK
JACOB J. SPIES

1

Overview

Peter D. Fox

That health care costs are rising rapidly is well known. However, the extent to which employers are either genuinely concerned with health care costs or willing to take action has been questioned. One widely quoted study concluded that business has only limited concerns (Sapolsky 1981). Whether that study represented an accurate interpretation of senior-level corporate attitudes at the time it was performed has been widely debated (Iglehart 1982). What is apparent is that these attitudes have changed dramatically since the beginning of the decade, reflecting annual premium increases that have commonly averaged 18 percent annually and, in many instances, have exceeded 30 percent.

Indeed, most employers and other purchasers—e.g., union management (Taft-Hartley) and multiemployer trust funds—have recently made commitments not to stand idly by as health care costs escalate, although many have yet to take forceful action. Others are just beginning to learn the complicated world of cost containment. Reflecting this resolve, the number of purchaser or purchaser-provider health care coalitions—local or regional organizations whose principal mission is cost containment—has more than doubled in the past year. Changes in plan design and new utilization review techniques that prevent the delivery of unnecessary care or care in an inappropriate setting are being adopted at an accelerated rate. The number of preferred provider organizations (PPOs), which use plan design incentives to encourage the use of efficient providers, that are in various stages of planning and development is many times the number that are in operation, signaling an upsurge in activity.

It is difficult to quantify the change in attitudes, short of formal, longitudinal surveys. One measure of the interest in cost containment is the growth in both staff numbers and salaries of health benefits managers, an indication that corporations are willing to "put their money where their mouth is." A few years ago, hardly any corporations had staffs devoted exclusively to health benefits; today quite a number have. Also, a 1982 survey of *Fortune* 1000 companies conducted by the Martin E. Segal Co. found that benefits managers are better compensated than before. Managers who responded to the survey reported an average annual salary of $45,000 in 1982, compared with $28,700 in 1978, a 57 percent increase, compared to the rise in wages of less than 30 percent for workers generally.

Federal and state governments are also reacting vigorously, and both the public and private sectors have demonstrated the value of learning from each other. More often than not, their actions are mutually reinforcing, notwithstanding arguments over whether one payer harms the other by causing providers to shift costs. For example:

— State governments and local planning agencies have stimulated the development of private coalitions (e.g., Utah, Colorado, South Florida), and some coalitions (e.g., Iowa, Toledo, Cleveland) are major actors in state health planning functions.

— Employers are increasingly contracting for utilization review (UR) with federally-funded peer review organizations as well as with other private review organizations that may, in the future, help the federal government assess the appropriateness of care provided to Medicare and Medicaid beneficiaries.

— Measures taken by the federal government to pay only what it defines as its fair share of costs have led, in the opinion of many, to the shifting of costs to the private sector. Whether or not this shifting is equitable, these measures have clearly been a major stimulant to private cost-containment activity.

This book provides an overview of the forces that underlie and stimulate changes, of the kinds of changes taking place, and of the possible implications of these changes. The topics and some of the key findings are as follows.

Benefits design

Many employers are seeking to increase and rationalize enrollee cost-sharing by reducing longstanding biases in benefit packages that favor institutional care. For example, more employers are applying cost-sharing to institutional services, adopting second opinion for surgery programs, and incorporating incentives to shift the locus of care from inpatient to outpatient settings. Some are also offering financial inducements for not using services and are beginning to manage their benefits in a more concerted way. They are, for example, channeling patients to efficient health care providers and assigning staff to do discharge planning for hospitalized employees and dependents in order to shorten length of stay. Other changes include allowing employees to select from among benefit packages and establishing individual medical expense accounts that employees can either use for medical expenses or receive as a cash payment.

Alternative delivery systems

Most employers and other purchasers have for some time been comfortable contracting with health maintenance organizations (HMOs), which has contributed to an annual growth in enrollment that has exceeded 10 percent for most of the last several years. More recently, purchasers, providers, and carriers have become excited about preferred provider organizations (PPOs), which incorporate incentives in the benefit package to encourage the use of selected providers, who in turn typically agree to discount their charges. One effect is the emergence of a spectrum of alternative delivery systems that embody a variety of risk sharing and organizational features and that do not fit neatly into boxes. Among the unanswered questions at this time are: the growth potential of PPOs and other new alternative delivery systems and the impact that they will have on the utilization of health services.

Utilization review

Utilization review, long thought necessary for Medicare but slow to develop in the private sector, is now the top priority of many employer cost-management strategies. It is of value in educational efforts with providers, in making decisions regarding whether to contract with particular PPOs, in structuring incentives for patients to use particular providers, and in benefit plan design. In its simplest form, UR simply identifies hospitalized patients who no longer have a medical reason to remain as inpatients. However, the scope of UR is being expanded to include prior authorization for hospitalization based upon model treatment plans, concurrent review of inpatient care, and the comparative analysis of hospital and physician performance. A new industry has emerged to analyze patient data and perform in-hospital UR for private payers.

Health care coalitions

In just the past three years, more than 100 states and local communities have organized coalitions—organizations whose specific focus is health care cost containment. The membership of some coalitions is restricted to purchasers; in others, providers participate as well. This development reflects the need for collective action as an essential component of cost-management strategies. The initial focus of coalitions, often, is mutual education. As coalitions mature, they typically create a broad-based community focus for health care management by venturing into such areas as data systems, utilization review, health planning, the development of alternative delivery systems, the promotion of wellness programs and community education, benefit redesign, and trustee education.

Worksite wellness programs

Worksite wellness programs are growing at a rapid pace, predicated upon the belief that health promotion activities will reduce medical expenditures, absenteeism, turnover, and accidents while increasing morale and productivity. Companies of all sizes are offering programs, some in-house and others through community resources such as the YMCA. Often focused on lifestyle changes that will reduce the risk of cardiovascular disease, the most common programs are smoking cessation, stress management, physical fitness, nutrition, weight control, and hypertension control. Increasingly, so-called employee assistance programs, aimed at helping overcome personal crises and substance abuse, have become part of corporate wellness programs. Evidence of their effectiveness is increasing, as are the numbers of programs, their comprehensiveness, and the extent of their integration with the other elements of employer cost-management strategies.

In-house corporate medical programs

As the corporation seeks to manage its benefits in a more focused way, the role of corporate medical departments will, of necessity, change as they participate in utilization review efforts, the analysis of medical data to assist in benefit plan design, and efforts to identify and encourage the use of efficient providers. In addition, a few companies have their own direct delivery programs. These companies typically provide primary care as a substitute for, or in addition to, coverage in the fee-for-service system and exert varying degrees of control over the provision of specialty and hospital care.

Hospital trustee activities

In some communities, hospital trustees have accepted cost containment as one of their missions and have promoted reforms in a number of ways. Some have focused on the management of their own institutions. Others have undertaken communitywide efforts, often through a local trustee council that they have formed. Trustees in some communities have also become active in designing and supporting legislative changes, such as state rate setting. In addition, some corporations have sought to ensure that employees who are members of hospital boards are equipped for that role and understand cost-containment issues. An important issue is the potential conflict between the trustee's role vis-à-vis the hospital and the cost-containment objectives of the corporation.

Purchaser cost-containment strategy

Many purchasers have found it desirable to evolve a multifaceted cost-management strategy rather than relying on a single approach. Such a strategy typically entails a combination of actions taken individually (e.g., benefit design changes), joint actions, often taken through local or regional coalitions (e.g., joint data analysis, utilization review, and community education), and actions to influence government (e.g., seeking to eliminate barriers to competition, promoting state rate setting, and participating in facilities planning).

Each of the above activities is discussed in the following chapters of this book. Taken together, they constitute a comprehensive description of the principal corporate efforts to control health care expenditures.

REFERENCES

Iglehart, J. K. "American Health Care and Business." *New England Journal of Medicine* 306(January 1982):120–24.

Sapolsky, H. M., D. Altman, R. Greene, and J. D. Moore. "Corporate Attitudes toward Health Care Costs." *Milbank Memorial Fund Quarterly* 59(Fall 1981):561–85.

2

Plan Design

Peter D. Fox

INTRODUCTION

For most large-group coverage, benefit payments account for more than 90 percent of the premium dollar. The remainder (the retention) pays the costs of administration and profit. Traditionally, private purchasers of care—e.g., single employers, multiemployer trusts, and union-management (Taft-Hartley) trusts—have concerned themselves predominantly with issues of retention rates and cash flow and have assumed a rather passive attitude towards the more than 90 percent of the health care dollar that is spent on benefits. Furthermore, a growing economy, the need to compete for skilled labor, and federal tax treatment of employer contributions to premiums all encouraged benefit expansions.

However, employers and unions have become increasingly interested in controlling the dollars spent on benefits. In doing so, they tend to focus naturally on plan design, since plan design issues are understandable, are under the discretion of the individual purchaser, and rarely entail direct confrontation with providers.

Rising benefit costs are the major reason for this focus. Between 1978 and 1980, only a two-year period, health care costs as a percent of payroll increased from 5.27 percent to 6.96 percent (HRI 1981). Between 1978 and 1981, premium increases averaged around 17 percent (NAEHCA 1983), and some firms witnessed increases in excess of 30 percent.

Another reason has been the need to adapt to a more complex environment. Until the 1960s, there were only a handful of prepaid group practices, and the carriers needed to recognize the existence mostly of hospitals and physicians. Thus, there were few ambiguities regarding the services and types of providers that were to be reimbursed.

In recent years, new delivery systems have come into existence. For example, the number of organizations that can be identified as prepaid group practices has expanded from 28 in 1970 to 265 in 1981 (Strumpf 1981, InterStudy 1983). It is likely that the remainder of this decade will witness further development of new organizational structures that may defy unambiguous definition. Preferred provider organizations and primary care networks, discussed in chapter 3, are examples of newly emerging plans.

In addition, new types of providers have either come into being or have become much more prevalent. Examples include freestanding ambulatory surgery units, freestanding emergicare or urgicare centers, nursing home care as a substitute for hospitalization, home health as a substitute for both nursing home and hospital services, hospice care, physician extenders and other mid-level practitioners, birthing centers, and various types of mental health personnel. The interest of the purchaser in broader coverage can stem from either a desire to create an improved program for enrollees or the belief that the new services are a substitute for more expensive services. One question that is inevitably raised is whether these services are truly substitutes or whether, instead, the total quantity of services purchased rises as a result of the increased capacity of the system to deliver them. In some cases, state law has required coverage, although, as discussed below, self-insuring plans are exempt from most state insurance laws as a consequence of the Employee Retirement Income Security Act of 1974 (ERISA).

Benefit design entails three principal sets of decisions:

— What services should be covered?
— What should be the cost-sharing and reimbursement structure, encompassing:
  — deductibles
  — coinsurance (the proportion of the bill that is paid by the enrollee)
  — copayments (a fixed amount per item of service, e.g., per doctor visit, per drug prescription, per day of hospitalization)
  — other reimbursement limitations
— What should be the premium share between employers and employees?

The focus of this chapter is on initiatives rather than on trends or changes. What constitutes an initiative is to some extent, like beauty, in the eye of the beholder. We have, for example, discussed evidence of increased cost-sharing, not because there is anything innovative about cost-sharing per se but because the move to increase cost-sharing represents a reversal of prior trends and because the range of implementation strategies is of interest.

The remaining sections of this chapter discuss cost-sharing, targeted measures to decrease hospital use, prudent purchasing, multiple choice indemnity plans, cash health incentive and medical expense accounts, and channeling.

Thoughtful purchasers are not making changes one at a time; rather, they are developing strategies that reflect not only what might be ideal but also corporate history and culture, employee and union relations, and other factors that are unique to their situation. They are also integrating plan design decisions with other efforts described in this report. This and other matters are discussed in the conclusion to this chapter. In addition, the appendix to this chapter summarizes the major benefit plan contracting mechanisms—i.e., experience rating, self-insurance, and minimum premium plans—for readers who are unfamiliar with the distinctions among them.

Throughout this chapter, specific examples of purchaser and carrier initiatives are cited. They are intended to be illustrative and are not an exhaustive compilation. Particularly in light of the high activity level, these examples could be expanded considerably.

This chapter reports statistics from a variety of surveys, specifically those of the Hay-Huggins Company; the National Association of Employers on Health Care Alternatives (NAEHCA); the Health Research Institute (HRI); Towers, Perrin, Forster, & Crosby (TPF&C); and the Mercer Company. All of these surveys were conducted in 1982, except for the Hay-Huggins survey, which was conducted in 1983, and HRI, which was conducted in 1981. In each case, the sample consists predominantly of large companies. The statistics reported are indicative only, for a variety of reasons. In several cases the response rate was below 40 percent. Most large companies with a multiplicity of unions and subsidiaries have a number of plans (quite a few have more than 100), and, typically, only one is reflected in a response. Some of the survey questions have elements of ambiguity. For example, a company, in responding to a question on whether it had a program to cover second opinions for surgery, might or might not respond affirmatively if it reimbursed for the office visit (which essentially all major medical plans do) but took no other actions to encourage second opinions. In addition, the surveys do not include Taft-Hartley or multiemployer trust funds, small or medium employers, or federal, state, or local employees. (However, the Office of the Assistant Secretary for Planning and Evaluation in the U.S. Department of Health and Human Services has funded the Hay-Huggins Company to expand its sample to include small employers and Taft-Hartley and multiemployer trust funds.)

COST-SHARING

Cost-sharing serves two functions. First, it shifts costs from the plan to the enrollee. Second, it creates incentives for enrollees to reduce their utilization by increasing out-of-pocket expenses (Newhouse 1981). Many existing plans favor the use of the inpatient setting by having lower cost-sharing for hospital, and commonly surgical, services. By increasing cost-sharing, the intent of most firms is not only to shift the burden to the employee but to redirect utilization to be more appropriate.

For purposes of this paper, cost-sharing initiatives are classified into two categories. The first, discussed in this section, relates to changes that apply to broad classes of services, such as all hospital services and/or all physician services. The second, discussed in the following section, entails changes in a more narrow set of services, typically designed to shift the locus of care to less expensive—predominantly nonhospital—settings.

Virtually all plans have cost-sharing to some degree. The historical trend since the introduction of health insurance has been to decrease out-of-pocket costs to enrollees by covering new services (e.g., outpatient physician services, drugs, and dental care), by decreasing coinsurance and deductibles, and by adding maximums on cost-sharing beyond which the plan pays in full. For example, according to the Hay-Huggins survey, 77 percent of group plans surveyed have a catastrophic, or stop-loss, provision that limits out-of-pocket expenses for coinsurance (typically in the $500–$1,000 range) that an individual must face; ten years ago, such a provision was rare. Similarly, today, almost all large group plans cover office visits; in 1975, 32 percent of plans did not cover physician office visits for employees, and 40 percent did not cover them for dependents. One way in which cost-sharing has been systematically reduced is in plans with deductibles that have remained constant over time, often at $50 per person annually. The result has been to improve benefits in real terms due to the effect of inflation.

It is our strong impression that purchasers are seeking to raise deductibles, although formal surveys show at most a weak effect, and only a minority of large purchasers have made changes. Hay-Huggins reports that, in 1983, 11 percent of employers surveyed had deductibles in excess of $100, compared to 2 percent in both 1979 and 1975. (The respondents to the Hay-Huggins survey change somewhat from year to year. About one-third are new each year, representing both client growth and turnover.) The proportion of firms with base plus supplemental major medical programs (as opposed to comprehensive major medical programs with cost-sharing on almost all services) increased from 67 percent in 1979 to 73 percent in 1981, and then declined to 62 percent in 1982.* Similarly HRI reports that, between 1979 and 1981, the proportion of companies with base plus supplemental major medical programs decreased from 69 percent to 61 percent, while the proportion of comprehensive major medical increased from 32 percent to 39 percent. Mercer reports that, in the last two years, 33 percent of responding companies raised their deductibles or established higher copayments.

These changes are not dramatic. However, from our interviews, we believe that they are symptomatic of an accelerating trend. We have also had access to the data files of Towers, Perrin, Forster, & Crosby, a large management and benefits consulting firm. They report that more than half of their large corporate clients that have made significant design changes in the last two years shifted from a base plan plus major medical to either a comprehensive major medical or a multiple option plan that included comprehensive major medical coverage as one of the offerings.

One of the most dramatic changes was at the Jones and Laughlin Steel Company, a subsidiary of LTV, which related cost-sharing to wages. (A number of companies relate premium contribution levels to wages. However, we do not know of any other plans, besides LTV and Xerox, described below, that have related cost-sharing to wages.) In January 1983, it introduced a per family annual deductible on all services, other than hospital services, equal to 1 percent of annualized wages. Thus an earner with $20,000 in earnings would face a $200 deductible per family, whereas a senior executive earning $100,-000 would face a $1,000 deductible. Expenses above the deductible are subject to 20 percent coinsurance, with a maximum on out-of-pocket expenses (deductible plus coinsurance) of 3 percent of wages. Previously, the cost-sharing structure included a $175 deductible and 20 percent coinsurance. However, a generous base program paid in full for all hospital and many physician services.

Xerox Corporation introduced a similar structure for its 45,000 salaried workers in January 1984, and the company is in the process

---

* A base ("basic") pays in full, in contrast to a major medical program that typically has a deductible and coinsurance. A common benefits structure is for hospital, surgical, and, sometimes, diagnostic services to be paid in full up to some level, with the excess covered by a supplemental major medical plan. The other common structure is a comprehensive major medical, which does not have a base program and thus has cost sharing on most, or all, services.

of negotiating this approach with its unionized workers, 5,000 of whom are in the new plan as of this writing. Previously, employees had a $100 per person deductible, with a maximum of $200 in deductible expenses per family, and payment-in-full for hospital and surgical expenses. Most other services were subject to 20 percent cost-sharing once expenses exceeded the deductible. Instead, the deductible is now 1 percent of pay (single deductible per family) and 20 percent coinsurance for most expenses above the deductible, including hospital and surgical services. An out-of-pocket maximum has been set at the lesser of 4 percent of pay or $4,000 a year, excluding psychiatric care, which will continue to have 50 percent cost-sharing and no limitation on out-of-pocket expenses.

In addition, Xerox has initiated medical expense accounts that it calls "flexible benefit accounts," to which the company plans to contribute $400 annually for each employee. A medical expense account is a separate account for each employee that can be drawn from to pay out-of-pocket medical expenses, including cost-sharing, the cost of uncovered services, and the employee's premium share. (Medical expense accounts are discussed below in more detail under "Financial Incentive Programs.") Any money that is not used for such expenses is, at the end of the year, either returned to the employee in cash or allowed to accumulate in the medical expense account. Although the tax status of this approach has not been definitely established, the company presumes that the portion of the account that is used for medical expenses is not taxable as income to the employee, whereas the amount paid out in cash is taxable. The company estimates that the $400 equates roughly to the savings that the plan would realize, assuming no change in use of medical services. The savings from lower utilization generated by the increased cost-sharing will accrue entirely to the company. Xerox estimates these savings at between 5 and 10 percent of premiums.

Xerox reports that the changes have met with less resistance than the company had anticipated. This is attributed in part to an extensive educational campaign that was mounted to inform the work force of the problems of rising health care costs and the need for the company to be competitive in the face of both domestic and foreign, especially Japanese, competition.

The Quaker Company adopted an innovative approach to implementing cost-sharing increases. Until January 1983, this company had a fairly standard base plus supplemental major medical, with payment in full for surgical expenses and for outpatient diagnostic expenses up to $200 and hospital expenses up to $6,000. The major medical plan, which reimbursed the excess over the base plan, plus a broad array of other services, had a $100 deductible (maximum of two per family) and 20 percent coinsurance.

Effective January 1983, the base program was eliminated, thereby subjecting all hospital, surgical, and diagnostic services to cost-sharing. The deductible was raised to $300 per employee unit (single or family coverage), with 85 percent payment (i.e., 15 percent coinsurance) on expenses above the deductible. In addition, $300 was given to each employee in the form of a medical expense account. This $300 roughly equals the savings that result from the higher cost-sharing structure, assuming no change in utilization. In fiscal year 1982, the company spent $1,367 per employee; for calendar year 1983, the company has promised its employees that it would contribute $1,535, a 12.3 percent increase over an 18-month period. If the cost of the health benefits, including the contribution to the medical expense accounts, averages less than $1,535, then the difference will be divided among employees in the form of additional contributions to their accounts. The presumption is that this difference would result from reduced utilization. By linking the additional contributions to utilization reductions of all employees, the company has created a group incentive to be cost-conscious.

From the Quaker Company's perspective, the approach has a number of attractive features. Because the savings resulting from the higher cost-sharing are distributed to employees through the medical expense account, and many do not use their health benefits, the majority of employees—i.e., those who consume few services—will be better off than before. More importantly, in future years, the company can target a percentage rate of increase. If actual expenditures exceed the target, there would be an offsetting reduction in the contribution to the medical expense account. (For 1984, an 8 percent increase is planned.) Thus, the program assumes some of the characteristics of a defined contribution, rather than a defined benefits, plan. The expectation is that the nature of negotiations with both salaried employees and union representatives will shift from focusing purely on benefit levels and will, instead, address the rate of increase in benefit payments. In addition, the company believes that healthy employees have disproportionately enrolled in HMOs and that the new plan will induce some of these to elect the indemnity plan instead because of its lower premiums. Finally, although it has not yet done so, the company plans to supplement this new approach with an effort to identify and encourage the use of efficient hospitals and doctors, similar to the channeling programs to be described. Thus, cost-sharing changes are being addressed in the context of an overall cost-management strategy, and the cost-sharing and medical expense account structures explicitly make employees partners in this effort. The concept of a cost-management strategy is discussed further in the concluding chapter of this book.

Other companies that have eliminated base programs have introduced some offsetting benefit improvements, most of which are designed to shift patterns of care to nonhospital settings. For example, Rockwell International and FMC Corporation recently eliminated their base programs and subjected most services, including hospital services, to 10 percent coinsurance. Previously, FMC had 15 percent and Rockwell International had 20 percent coinsurance in their major medical plans. Thus, the 10 percent coinsurance represents a benefit reduction in hospital benefits and an improvement for major medical expenses. However, both companies continue to exempt from cost-sharing a few services that are intended principally to shift care from inpatient to outpatient settings. Rockwell International exempts preadmission testing, birthing clinic services, ambulatory surgery, and both second opinions for surgery and the surgery itself if the second opinion confirmed the need. It projects a savings of 12 percent overall on its plan as a result of these changes. FMC exempted outpatient lab and x-ray, ambulatory surgery, preadmission testing, skilled nursing facility (SNF) and home health care, birthing clinic services, and hospice care.

Other companies have eliminated the base program with, at most, minor offsetting improvements. Boise Cascade, for example, did so and also increased the deductible from $100 to $150 per person, although this company, too, pays in full for a small handful of services in order to reduce inpatient care (e.g., preadmission testing, ambulatory surgery, home health, and second surgical opinions). Like most companies, it mounted a major educational campaign to inform employees about rising health care costs and the need for change. There was some surprise at the low level of negative reaction expressed by the salaried employees affected. Similar changes are being negotiated in the company's union plans.

In addition to changes in programs of large employers, a number of joint union-management trust funds, such as those in the construction trades, that receive fixed, negotiated cents-per-hour contributions for health benefits, have recently introduced coinsurance in lieu of base programs.

Some carriers are also promoting higher cost-sharing. Ironically, they appear to be doing so mostly for large, experience-rated companies, rather than small groups, where they are at risk. Examples of changes directed towards large groups include the "cost fighter" program that Lincoln National has begun to market. One feature is that enrollees pay the room and board charges for the first day in the hospital, unless medical testing was performed prior to admission. Lincoln National proposes to pay only 80 percent of charges through the 14th day of hospitalization but 100 percent thereafter. It is also proposing to pay 80 percent of surgical fees. Aetna is promoting comprehensive major medical coverage with a $200 per person deductible and 20 percent coinsurance with a maximum limit on coinsurance of $1,000. Prudential has also significantly increased its deductibles for its small groups.

In addition, some Blue Cross and Blue Shield plans are promoting the so-called health credit concept, which removes from the provider the onus of collecting cost-sharing. Under this approach, the provider bills and receives full payment from either the plan or a bank with which the plan contracts. The plan or the bank, in turn, collects applicable cost-sharing from the patient, with the employer typically being at risk ultimately for any bad debts. This allows the Blues to continue to pay providers in full and, at the same time, introduce cost-sharing. (In some cases, the doctor may collect a small co-payment directly from the patient.) It also significantly reduces paperwork for providers. The largest such programs are at Kodak and Xerox in Rochester, New York. Kodak reports that it has experienced only minimal bad debts. (The Xerox plan has insufficient experience to report as of this writing.) Other Blue Cross plans that have adopted the same concept are those in New Jersey and Michigan.

Some coalitions have developed model benefit packages that are intended to promote cost-sharing. For example, provisions of the model plan of the Birmingham (Alabama) coalition, aspects of which have been adopted by several of its member companies (e.g., South Central Bell, Gulf States Paper), include the following. Employees pay the room and board charges for the first day of hospitalization and $25 a day for the second through the tenth. They are also responsible for the full costs incurred on Friday or Saturday for admissions on those days, unless the illness is of an emergency nature or the hospital has weekend diagnostic workers. Outpatient diagnostic services are paid in full, whether or not they are associated with a hospitalization, but inpatient diagnostic services are paid at 80 percent. Surgery is reimbursed at 90 percent if a second opinion was obtained, and 50 percent if it was not. In addition, the coalition is experimenting with a global fee program that would reimburse physicians on a per case basis, whether the services are performed in or out of the hospital.

The South Florida Health Action Coalition is also actively promoting changes in benefit design. It has developed a comprehensive benefits matrix that in effect creates a comprehensive major medical, with coinsurance applied to all but a few services, such as hospice care.

TARGETED MEASURES TO DECREASE HOSPITAL USE

Purchasers are well aware that hospital services are the most expensive part of the benefit package. As a result, in addition to imposing cost-sharing on hospital services, some are incorporating other provisions that are designed mostly to shift the locus of care to ambulatory settings. In some instances, cost savings have not been clearly documented, and the changes could potentially increase cost, depending on how the program is structured and managed. Indeed, it is the willingness to manage selected benefits—including communicating and negotiating with enrollees and providers, rather than simply establishing payment rules and processing claims—that is likely to characterize a successful cost-containment strategy. This distinction is relevant to the discussion in this section on preadmission testing, home health benefits, and prior authorization, and to the section on channeling as well.

The plan design features examined in this section are second opinion for surgery, ambulatory surgery, preadmission testing, and convalescent benefits. One other measure relates to weekend admissions. Some companies will not pay for Friday, Saturday, or Sunday admissions unless they are medically justified. For example, FMC Corporation has introduced such a limitation.

Second Opinions for Surgery

Virtually all major medical plans reimburse an enrollee who obtains a second opinion for surgery, which for claims processing purposes may be indistinguishable from any other office visit, as part of the major medical benefit package. More recently, purchasers have actively begun to promote second opinions.

In designing a second opinion program that extends beyond simply reimbursing the cost of the office visit and associated lab tests, the purchaser faces a number of decisions. The reimbursement level for the second opinion must be determined. Many plans waive the usual cost-sharing and, instead, pay in full. As to the source of the second opinion, most plans allow the enrollee to obtain the second opinion from any physician or, alternatively, any physician qualified to perform the surgery. Less commonly, a panel of physicians is established. One concern with a program without a panel is that the primary surgeon will often be the source of referral to the doctor who renders the second opinion, and the second doctor may be loath to question the judgment of the referring docor. Another concern is that many patients may have difficulty responding to the intent of the program without some assistance and direction, which a defined panel offers.

Questions also arise as to the extent of promotional efforts. The key to a successful second opinion program is an active employee educational and communication effort.

A decision must be made establishing the consequences of failing to obtain a second opinion. The available options are to have a totally voluntary program, with no penalties or rewards; to have cost-sharing incentives or disincentives, either for all nonemergency procedures or for a selected list of procedures; or to have a mandatory program that does not pay any benefits if a second opinion has not been obtained, either for all nonemergency procedures or for a selected list. In the event of a negative second opinion, what will the reimbursement status be under incentive or mandatory programs? Most such programs will not apply cost-sharing penalties if the second opinion is negative and the surgery is obtained anyway. Many also encourage enrollees to seek a third opinion.

The prevalence of second opinion programs is not known with great accuracy, although it is clearly on the rise. HRI reports that 67 percent of companies surveyed will pay for a second opinion (an increase from 52 percent in 1979), 47 percent actively encourage obtaining second opinions, and 2 percent have incentive or mandatory programs. In the NAEHCA survey, 55 percent of respondents reported having programs in 1982, compared with 37.5 percent in 1980. Finally, Hay-Huggins reports that 8 percent have mandatory or incentive programs.

Thus, most second surgical opinion programs are voluntary. However, increasingly, purchasers are establishing lists of procedures that have high nonconfirmation rates (the percent of second opinions that do not confirm the first surgeon's recommendation for surgery) and are applying a cost-sharing penalty if a second opinion is not obtained. For example, they will apply 50 percent coinsurance in a plan that would otherwise have 20 percent coinsurance, or introduce 20 percent coinsurance in a plan that would otherwise pay in full. To illustrate, starting January 1983, Owens-Illinois, for 13 procedures, pays 100 percent reimbursement if a second opinion is obtained but only 80 percent of both the surgeon's fee and hospitalization if it is not. May D & F, a department store chain in Denver, in its coverage through Metropolitan Life Insurance Company, introduced a flat $200 copayment penalty where the second opinion is not obtained. The company reasoned that the $200 copayment is simpler and more visible than a coinsurance penalty.

Among the commercial carriers, Prudential pioneered second opinion programs, which it both markets actively to its large groups and includes within the benefits plan for its own employees. It offers both voluntary and incentive programs. Under the incentive plan, for a given list of procedures, if a second opinion is not confirmed, Prudential pays either 50 percent in a plan that normally would pay 80 percent of charges, or 80 percent in a plan that would pay 100 percent. Importantly, Prudential has enlisted a panel of nearly 20,000 board-certified physicians nationwide to provide second opinions. Panel members agree not to perform the surgery themselves. Prudential will apply cost-sharing penalties if the second opinion is negative and will also pay for a third opinion, plus any necessary x-ray and lab services.

Prudential originally required the second opinion for 506 procedures but has now reduced the number to 114, falling into 14 large diagnostic categories.

Prudential's categories are:

— hysterectomy

— cholecystectomy

— herniorrhaphy

— intervertebral disc or spinal surgery

— tonsillectomy and/or adenoidectomy

— prostatectomy

— cataract removal

— hemorrhoidectomy

— varicose vein ligation

— deviated septum (non-cosmetic)

— tympanotomy

— appendectomy (non-emergency)

— tubes and ovaries (non-obstetrical and non-sterilization)

— joint surgery (arthrectomies, arthrotomies and arthroplasties)

This approach is illustrative of programs that are limited to selected procedures.

Prudential reports that roughly 10 to 15 percent of the large groups it covers have adopted the second opinion program. Of those, some 80 percent have selected the incentive program, and 20 percent the voluntary program. The company is convinced that savings result. Premium reductions are offered of 2 percent for programs that reduce reimbursement from 100 percent to 80 percent, and 4 percent for programs that reduce reimbursement from 80 percent to 50 percent. Several other insurance companies—e.g., Aetna, Travelers, John Hancock—have incentive second opinion programs, usually for selected procedures, and self-funded employers have introduced them as well. CIGNA, another commercial carrier, offers voluntary programs only but does have panels of doctors in areas of high enrollment concentration who will give second opinions.

A less common variant of cost-sharing differentials involves rewards instead of penalties. For example, Rockwell International has a comprehensive major medical program with 10 percent coinsurance on most services. However, if a second opinion is obtained for any of 22 surgical procedures, the enrollee is reimbursed 100 percent of the cost of both the second opinion and the surgery.

Few private programs are totally mandatory, and these are mostly limited to union plans, such as the storeworkers and the building service workers unions in New York. Beginning in 1972, the Cornell University–New York Hospital helped several Taft-Hartley trust funds establish mandatory programs. (Under these programs, each family covered is forgiven once if a member of the family had surgery performed without obtaining a second opinion.) Cornell researchers found that the mandatory program saved $2.63 for every dollar spent. The researchers have also concluded that the benefit-to-cost ratio would have been higher if the covered procedures had been limited to a select list (Finkel et al. 1981).

In addition to these private programs, seven states have adopted mandatory second opinion programs in their Medicaid programs. Most of these programs require a second opinion for a select list of procedures. Although the population covered under Medicaid may not be directly comparable to a private pay population, utilization results have been very similar to studied private programs. Results from Massachusetts, Michigan, and Wisconsin indicate that these mandatory programs may have benefit-to-cost ratios of 2:1 or greater (Roenigk and Bartlett 1982).

Several conclusions may be drawn from the accumulated experience of private programs, union plans, Medicaid, and Medicare. First, few eligibles obtain second opinions under totally voluntary programs—usually less than 3 percent of the enrollees (Friedlob 1982, Joffe et al. 1980). Second, nonconfirmation rates in voluntary programs normally range from 25 to 35 percent among enrollees who do obtain second opinions, while in mandatory programs nonconfirmation rates typically range from 15 to 25 percent. The higher nonconfirmation rates in voluntary programs are probably due to the self-selection of patients who are more uncertain about having surgery performed (Finkel et al. 1981, Poggio et al. 1981). Third, the percentage of nonconfirmed patients who elect to undergo surgery is usually 30 to 50 percentage points less than the confirmed group. Some have suggested that a confirming opinion may increase the likelihood of surgery and thus increase the overall surgery rate, since confirmations outnumber nonconfirmations. However, experience from mandatory programs has usually shown a decrease in the overall surgery rate of between 5 and 15 percent (Roenigk et al. 1982, Poggio et al. 1981).

The evidence also indicates that the potential cost savings from a second opinion program are dependent on the nature and design of the program. Voluntary programs are likely to achieve only minimal cost savings due to low participation rates and fixed costs for program operation. Properly designed mandatory programs do yield cost savings. Little information exists about the cost savings potential of incentive/disincentive programs (Galblum 1980, Finkel et al. 1981).

Ambulatory Surgery

Developments in ambulatory surgery represent a classic case of a new form of practice and the need for insurance coverage to adapt. Ambulatory surgery can be performed in three settings: the hospital outpatient department, a freestanding ambulatory surgery center (FSASC), and the doctor's office. The physician's fee is covered in all three settings, and it is the reimbursement for the use of the facility that has been problematic to varying degrees. In the doctor's office, the physician's fee is usually assumed to include associated overhead expenses, although whether it really does so adequately for procedures that might be performed in other settings has been questioned. Hospital outpatient services have tended to be adequately covered. The area that has raised the most controversy in recent years has been coverage of FSASCs.

FSASCs arose initially in Arizona and Rhode Island around 1970. The Freestanding Ambulatory Surgical Association reports that in 1983 there were roughly 125 facilities that could be classified as FSASCs. The first comprehensive study of their cost was conducted under a contract with the Department of Health, Education, and Welfare (HEW) in 1977 (Orkand 1977). For the procedures studied, it found the facility fee for surgery in hospital outpatient departments to be 55 percent less than that for inpatient care. It also found services in FSASCs to be less expensive than in hospital outpatient departments.

Currently, most plans recognize FSASCs, although some Blue Cross plans have been slow to certify them. HRI reports that 92 percent of employers surveyed cover ambulatory surgery. Some plans, including commercial and self-insured ones, will pay the hospital bill in full but apply coinsurance to hospital outpatient department or FSASC charges, thereby encouraging high cost inpatient care.

As a result, many purchasers have sought to correct these biases. In addition, some actively encourage ambulatory over inpatient surgery, in one of four ways. First, some plans will pay at a higher level for selected procedures if they are performed on an ambulatory basis. For example, Rockwell International, which has a comprehensive major medical program with 10 percent coinsurance, will waive that coinsurance for selected procedures that are performed on an ambulatory basis. Owens-Illinois, which normally pays in full, will pay only 80 percent of the surgeon's fee and hospital expenses for surgery that could be performed on an outpatient basis. Unlike Rockwell International, Owens-Illinois does not specify in advance the procedures or circumstances under which the lower reimbursement applies.

Second, a few plans have adopted incentives for physicians. For example, May D & F department stores in Denver, under a plan with Metropolitan Insurance Company, has a list of procedures for which the surgeon will be paid 25 percent more if surgery is performed on an ambulatory basis than if it is performed in a hospital. Blue Cross of Michigan, under some of its plans, will pay 25 percent more than the usual and customary reimbursement level for 26 specific procedures if performed on an outpatient basis, and 25 percent less if performed on an inpatient basis. Also, under an 18-month pilot program initiated by Blue Cross of North Carolina, 88 procedures have been identified that can be performed in a doctor's office. The physician is reimbursed an additional 25 percent if the procedure is, in fact, performed in the office. This program was initiated in part out of concern that the growth in ambulatory surgery centers would encourage services being performed in these centers rather than in the office.

The third approach is prior authorization for selected procedures. These programs typically address the locus of care rather than the necessity of the procedure. Thus, a hysterectomy would not be questioned because it is not a candidate for being performed on an outpatient basis. Philadelphia Blue Cross introduced a prior authorization requirement for inpatient removal of impacted teeth, resulting in a shift from 80 percent of such procedures being performed on an inpatient basis to 80 percent being performed on an outpatient basis. Other procedures will be added to the program. Colorado Blue Shield and Blue Cross, working with the Colorado Foundation for Medical Care, developed a list of 55 procedures for which prior authorization is required, and they are planning to expand this list.

The final approach is through informational campaigns. For example, Blue Cross of North Carolina has initiated a major campaign directed at providers and employers. Between 1978 and 1982, for seven classes of procedures examined, this effort, combined with plan design changes, resulted in an increase in the proportion of surgeries performed on an outpatient basis from 25 percent to 38 percent.

As with second opinion for surgery, a properly designed program to promote ambulatory surgery can generate savings, although the magnitude of the savings is difficult to estimate. Some caveats are in order, however, that indicate the need for the carrier or purchaser to monitor the program carefully. First, in some cases, the facility fee can be very high, even above the costs of inpatient care. Second, the growth in ambulatory surgery units may result in the promotion of more surgery through supply-induced demand. It may also result in the shifting of the locus of some surgical procedures from the less expensive doctor's office. Finally, the development of ambulatory surgery centers in the absence of bed and other facility reductions may yield higher health system costs, although individual purchasers who shift the locus of care may realize savings.

Preadmission Testing

Preadmission testing is one benefit design change for which rhetoric has outstripped reality. It is a classic situation in which a design change in the absence of a process for managing the benefits can increase costs, and the purchaser may never know whether it did or not. The prevalence of preadmission testing provisions is not reported here because of concerns we have about the reliability of the questions in the various surveys.

The principal reason for covering preadmission testing is to discourage patients from being admitted to the hospital earlier than necessary. The problem was particularly severe at a time when many plans covered only inpatient services, and major medical plans were less common than they are today. Many plans still have cost-sharing arrangements that retain a bias towards inpatient care by paying in full in the hospital but not on a preadmission basis. However, increasingly, many plans do just the reverse; in the interest of achieving cost savings, they pay in full for preadmission testing, even though other services are subject to coinsurance.

However, the intended cost savings may not result. A few hospitals will repeat the tests anyway, and only rarely will hospitals accept tests performed at another facility or in the doctor's office. A related problem is that some hospitals have internal policies dictating that they perform certain tests on all patients, regardless of the reason for admission. This practice is a questionable one. For example, the routine taking of x-rays had more justification when tuberculosis was prevalent, yet some hospitals still require the routine performance of x-rays. As a final caveat, it is important to recognize that most hospital bills do not itemize the specific tests that are performed and, hence, the payer may not know whether tests were repeated.

A few employers have taken the initiative of meeting with representatives of those hospitals that their employees use most frequently to review their internal scheduling procedures and obtain assurances that tests performed outside of the hospital within a given time of admission (e.g., two weeks) will be accepted as valid and not repeated. An even smaller number of employers (e.g., Rohr Industries in San Diego) have negotiated changes in the scheduling procedures of hospitals and physicians so that where inpatient testing is appropriate, the surgery can be performed on the same day as the testing.

Blue Cross of Philadelphia has adopted a somewhat different approach. It pays a bonus of between five dollars and eight dollars to hospitals for each battery of tests performed on a preadmission basis. Its contracts with the hospital specify that the tests not be repeated. Although the patient bill does not provide sufficient information to disclose whether tests have been repeated, the medical records are spot checked if a problem is suspected. The plan is trying to negotiate reciprocity arrangements so that hospitals will accept each other's tests.

Convalescent Benefits

Convalescent benefits include home health services, either by a visiting nurse directly or through a home health agency; skilled nursing facility (SNF) services; and hospice care. The home health and SNF benefits are typically directed at patients in an acute or post-acute phase of illness rather than those in need of custodial care and are typically similar to those in Medicare. NAEHCA reports that 32 percent of its respondents cover home health services. It also reports that 36 percent cover SNF care. In contrast, Hay-Huggins estimates the prevalence of SNF coverage at 76 percent. Finally, NAEHCA estimates that 12 percent—and HRI, 13 percent—of plans cover hospice care.

Purchasers have two reasons for covering these benefits. The first is to improve coverage by encouraging access to care in the most appropriate setting, without necessarily having savings as an objective. The second is to achieve savings by substituting for more expensive hospital care. Some employers pay for home health and SNF services at 100 percent, even though other services, including inpatient services, are subject to coinsurance. In practice, these benefits tend not to be heavily utilized by the under-age-65 population, so that the cost impact is small. However, available evidence for home health and SNF care suggests that providing coverage in the absence of an effort to manage the care will cost rather than save money (DHHS 1981, Weissert et al. 1980).

An exciting development is the willingness of some plans to manage their convalescent benefits actively. Prudential has started an innovative program for home health benefits in Denver, Reno, and Las Vegas, named the patient management service. In each of the three cities, a nurse has been hired to visit hospitalized enrollees to determine if home health services might serve to shorten the length of stay. If the potential exists, the nurse will talk to the attending physician. Prudential has found that these physicians are often unaware of the home health benefit or how the services can be used. They report savings of $540,000 in 1983, less the cost of the three nurses plus associated overhead, and are considering expanding the program to other areas where they have high penetration.

In addition, a number of Blue Cross plans are actively promoting home health services as a way of reducing maternity costs, which commonly account for more than 10 percent of all benefit payments. For example, Blue Cross of Philadelphia will pay for up to three home health nurse visits and two homemaker/aide visits for new mothers who go home within 24 hours. This plan provision is intended to encourage the use of freestanding birthing centers or hospital birthing rooms followed by quick discharge. For new mothers discharged from the hospital within 24 hours, the Blue Cross plan in Rochester, New York, will provide three days of "family centered care," consisting of various in-home services, through the Genessee Region Home Care Association. These services are estimated to cost $70 per day, compared with $300 per day in the hospital. Finally, Blue Cross and Blue Shield of New Hampshire–Vermont has developed an arrangement with Concord Hospital in Manchester, New Hampshire. New mothers who are discharged within 24 hours of delivery are entitled to three nurse visits and three homemaker visits from designated visiting nurse associations.

PRUDENT PURCHASING

In the context of health benefits, prudent purchasing usually connotes negotiated or preset price arrangements entailing discounts or negotiated prices in situations where a retail outlet deals directly with the plan enrollee. Its most common application is in covering outpatient prescription drug and vision care benefits, although the concept could be expanded to other services as well, such as medical equipment and supplies. In addition to these kinds of arrangements, a few employers have independently negotiated discounts with hospitals that their employees use. For example, Rohr Industries in San Diego was able to negotiate discounts with local hospitals, and Gates Rubber Company in Denver receives roughly a 15 percent discount from Mercy Hospital and incorporates financial incentives in its plan design for employees to use the hospital.

Rockwell International in Cedar Rapids, Iowa, established its own pharmacy after it was unable to evolve satisfactory arrangements with local retail outlets. In 1979, it agreed to pay members of its major union the full cost of drugs, a benefit that was extended to salaried workers as well. In the view of the company, local pharmacies increased their prices as a result. When both the state and county pharmaceutical associations failed to respond with an acceptable approach, the company established its own pharmacy, with outlets at several plant locations. Ninety-six percent of all prescriptions are filled through the company pharmacy although its use is voluntary. The advantages to the employee include convenience and not having to file claims. The company estimates that it fills 400 prescriptions daily and realizes a net saving of almost $3.50 per prescription. It is now assessing other ways to channel patients to efficient providers and believes that the forceful action it took on its drug benefits increased its credibility with the local medical community regarding its seriousness of intent in achieving cost savings.

Another approach entails the use of mail-order drug companies. For example, the Manville Corporation in Denver, which has a standalone drug benefit, has an agreement with a mail-order company that sells drugs roughly at a wholesale price. Whereas prescriptions filled at a retail outlet are subject to 25 percent coinsurance, enrollees do not face cost-sharing, except for a small shipping fee, for drugs purchased through the mail. Similarly, the Pennsylvania state employees union has a contract with Thrift Drugs. Employees who order by mail are relieved of the one-dollar copay that otherwise applies. Generic drugs are substituted unless the prescription has an indication to the contrary. Thrift Drugs also maintains computer files that allow the checking of potentially dangerous cross-effects of multiple drugs. An estimated four dollars are saved for each prescription filled by mail.

Similar kinds of prudent purchasing arrangements have been negotiated for vision care. The purchaser or carrier develops price agreements with selected outlets. Enrollees may be required to use those outlets to receive a covered benefit, or the program may reimburse for items purchased elsewhere, but usually with higher cost-sharing. In some cases, vision care centers have been established rather than arrangements being negotiated with existing optometric outlets. For example, the Martin E. Segal Company, a benefits consulting firm, has done so on behalf of multiemployer trusts that are its clients. Finally, a few companies, e.g., Control Data Corporation in Minneapolis, have negotiated arrangements for discounted vision care, even though vision care is not part of their insurance program. The employee pays in full, but at a discounted rate.

MULTIPLE CHOICE INDEMNITY PLANS AND "CAFETERIA" BENEFITS

The concept of allowing employees to select among more than one indemnity plan, typically with differing levels of cost-sharing, has existed for a long time. The largest, and one of the oldest, examples is the Federal Employee Health Benefits Program. In the last few years, a small but growing number of companies have expanded their health benefits offerings to include more than one indemnity option.

Some of this growth has occurred in the context of "cafeteria," or flexible, benefits. Under the usual dual or multiple choice approach, the employee who selects a low-option plan pays less than one who elects a high-option. From a health insurance perspective, the major distinction of cafeteria benefits is that employees can apply the employer-contributed difference between the high- and low-option premium contribution towards a series of other benefits, such as various forms of insurance or contributions to savings accounts or retirement funds. Many of these benefits are either not subject to personal income tax or are tax-sheltered, meaning that taxes are typically deferred until a later date. This type of plan was initiated in the early 1970s. In 1974, ERISA effectively halted the development of such plans by construing the entire employer contribution as taxable income if the employee had the option of allocating any portion of that contribution to taxable benefits. This provision was changed in 1978, resulting in renewed interest, although some tax issues remain unresolved, which has caused many companies to hesitate. Among the first major companies to adopt cafeteria benefits were American Can, TRW, and Educational Testing Service.

Employers have several motives for offering cafeteria benefits. The first is that employees like being able to tailor the employer's contribution to meet their individual needs. One important impact in the health area relates to the growing number of two-earner families with access to duplicate coverage. If only one company has a cafeteria plan, the spouse employed by that company is likely to use the flexibility to purchase benefits other than health insurance, thereby loading the full cost of health coverage onto the other spouse's employer. Second, the amount of the employer contribution to benefits becomes more visible, since employees are more aware of the amount they have to allocate. Third, cafeteria plans may limit employer costs in the long run because the employer typically agrees to a contribution level rather than to pay for a defined set of health benefits, whose costs have historically risen at a rate that exceeds cost-of-living increases.

However, cafeteria plans do have drawbacks. First, they are more difficult to administer than traditional benefit programs and are more prone to employee misunderstanding, even with extensive communication efforts. Second, they can generate adverse selection, i.e., less healthy employees who anticipate having a high claims experience will be more willing to pay for better coverage than those who anticipate submitting few claims, thereby driving up the cost of the more comprehensive options. Third, employees whose benefit plans previously required contributions may find cafeteria plans sufficiently more attractive that they newly enroll, thereby increasing employer costs. For example, if the cafeteria offering includes a non-contributory low-option health benefits plan, whereas the previous plan required an employee contribution, some employees (particularly those with access to coverage through a working spouse) will enroll for the first time. Finally, some employees may make poor choices. This problem can be partially overcome by having a common (or core) set of benefits that all employees must accept, thereby assuring minimum levels of protection.

One other effect relates to HMOs. For employers with paid-in-full health insurance benefits, the HMO premium may be below the employer contribution to the competing conventional insurance plan, even though the conventional plan may have less comprehensive benefits. A cafeteria plan allows an HMO enrollee to apply the difference to other benefits, thereby making enrollment more attractive. (A cash rebate serves the same function. However, few employers offer cash rebates where the HMO premium is below the contribution to the indemnity plan.) This phenomenon benefits the HMO. On the other hand, the HMO is likely to have higher premiums than a low-option plan and face adverse selection as a result.

Leaving aside cafeteria plans, the most common reason for offering multiple indemnity options stems from the desire of employees for comprehensive coverage counterbalanced by the employers' interest in limiting costs. Less commonly, employers have offered multiple options as part of a strategy of reducing present or future benefits. For example, it has been used to achieve a transition from a base plus supplemental major medical program, which becomes the high option, to a comprehensive major medical program, which becomes the low option (e.g., Crown Zellerbach). One employer (B.F. Goodrich) instituted medical expense accounts (see next section) with a contribution set at the value of the difference between the contribution to the old indemnity plan and the new low option. Employees can apply their accounts towards the purchase of a medium or high option or, instead, retain it in the account.

Perhaps the most critical issue in structuring multiple indemnity offerings is the manner in which the employee contribution to the various plans is structured. Most employers offer two options, although some (e.g., American Can) have offered as many as five. The high option can be expected to cost more than the low option, due to the more comprehensive coverage and because of adverse selection. The extent of adverse selection differs among plans in ways that are not totally predictable and is an important topic that warrants further research.

The first decision facing employers concerns whether each option should be self-supporting, with employees paying the full difference in the per enrollee experience of the two options or, instead, whether to pool the experience to counter the effect of adverse selection. Some employers separately experience-rate each option (e.g., DuPont, Sun Oil). Many (e.g., Texaco, Hartford National Bank) have separately experience-rated initially—in some cases not anticipating adverse selection—and then have pooled the risk after adverse selection occurred. Others (e.g., J.C. Penney) anticipated the potential for adverse selection and pooled from the start. Still others have consciously used multiple choice offerings to drive up the price of the high option in order, ultimately, to eliminate it by making it so costly that few employees join. The adverse selection can create a premium spiral whereby, each year, the employee population that remains in the high option is less and less healthy, generating further disenrollment and ultimately driving the high option out of existence. Thus, multiple choice can serve as a way of achieving a transition from a base plus major medical (high option) to a comprehensive major medical structure (low option). Where the risks have been pooled, the employee contribution for those who select the high option is typically set to approximate the actuarial value of the difference between two benefit packages, i.e., to reflect the difference that would have resulted had identical populations enrolled in each plan.

FINANCIAL INCENTIVE PROGRAMS

In an effort to encourage employees to limit utilization, several employers are using financial incentives to reduce medical claims. One of the innovations that is being adopted at a fast pace is an approach that is known by a number of names: medical expense account, employee spending account, salary reduction plan, medical reimbursement plan, flexible benefit account, and so forth. (Among the companies with medical expense accounts are the Quaker Company, Alcoa, Mellon Bank, Berol, Chemical Bank, Comerica Bank, PepsiCo, LTV, Xerox, and Northern States Power).

The medical expense account, as described under Cost-Sharing in the discussion of the Xerox Company program, is an individual account for each participating employee that can be drawn from to pay out-of-pocket medical expenses, including cost-sharing, the cost of uncovered services, and employee premium contributions. Depending on the particular plan, it may also be used for certain other expenses that are not taxed or are tax deferred if paid by the employer, such as work-related dependent child care and disability premiums. Moneys for the medical expense accounts can be contributed either by the employer or through voluntary salary deductions. Under some plans, the monies remaining in the account at the end of the year are returned to the employee, whereas in others, the employee can elect whether to withdraw the balance or allow it to accumulate.

A closely related approach is the zero-balance reimbursement account (ZEBRA) under which, instead of being funded prospectively, the account is in effect funded at the time evidence of an expense is presented. The employee who submits the claim receives two checks, one for the amount of the claim and a payroll check that is reduced by that amount. Thus, the total employer liability is unchanged, since the sum of the two checks is the same (although savings in payroll taxes may be realized). Importantly, income and Social Security taxes are taken only out of the payroll check and not out of the medical expense check, thereby increasing the employee's after-tax income. Companies that have adopted this approach include Savannah Foods in Atlanta and Lewin and Associates in Washington.

The main impetus behind medical expense accounts is the tax treatment. Although still in a gray zone because the Internal Revenue Service has yet to issue a definitive ruling, lawyers have been willing to write opinion letters stating that medically related expenses charged against the accounts are not subject to personal income tax. However, in early 1984, the IRS did issue a press release stating that medical expenditures through medical expense accounts as commonly structured, particularly the ZEBRA accounts, were not exempt from personal income tax. The position in that press release has been challenged by many large corporations with regard to both the substance and the process for setting tax policy, and at the time of this writing the ultimate outcome is uncertain.

This approach is often combined with the introduction of higher cost sharing and labeled a financial incentive program to promote healthy behavior, in that the cost sharing is a deterrent to the use of services and, therefore, an incentive to stay well. However, few would justify cost-sharing, whatever its merits, as an incentive not to get sick. In fact, the major impetus is the tax treatment. The medical expense accounts in effect become a way of making an additional portion of employee income free from personal income (and Social Security) taxes, at essentially no cost to the firm.

In addition to individual incentives, some companies have introduced group incentives (the Quaker Company combined both individual and group incentives), and still others have introduced incentives related to specific medical services. As each of the programs tends to be unique, seven approaches that have received widespread attention are discussed below. Incentives to encourage health promotion or wellness activities are discussed in chapter 6 on wellness.

The Mendocino County Stay Well Programs–
Health Incentive Plan

The Stay Well Program began in 1979 as a response by the Mendocino County School District to possible budget cuts and rising health insurance premiums. It was designed jointly with Blue Shield of California to provide employees with financial incentives to reduce utilization and is one of the original medical expense account programs. Using the money budgeted for health insurance, the school set aside $500 for each participating employee and, with the remaining budget, contracted out with Blue Shield for a $500 deductible major medical policy. Employees also receive educational material about health promotion and wellness.

The important feature of the Mendocino Stay Well plan is that, if an employee's claims in a given year total less than $500, the unused portion of the employee's account accumulates and is given to the employee upon termination of employment. Thus, an employee who worked for ten years and did not file any claims could receive $5,000. This program has several advantages: first-dollar coverage is maintained, employees have a strong incentive to reduce medical claims, and the county earns interest on the unused self-insured fund.

In response to widespread interest, Blue Shield of California has begun to offer the program, now called the Health Incentive Plan, to other employers. Approximately 90 groups and 100,000 people are participating. In order to accommodate different needs, more than 15 variations of the plan have been offered. One of the more common changes from the program described above calls for a contribution to the account of $300 for individual employees and $500 for families. Also common is a provision by which the employee receives the unused portion of his account at the end of each year rather than upon termination of employment, thus providing a more immediate incentive to the employee.

The small size of the original program in the Mendocino County school district (200–400 employees) made an evaluation difficult. However, the county and other groups offering the program have noted high employee interest. In addition to reducing medical utilization, the program may be encouraging employees to use the insurance of a spouse. In 1982, Blue Shield, funded by the John A. Hartford Foundation, initiated a three-year evaluation of the Stay Well–Health Incentive Plan that will include an examination of utilization, health care costs, and employee absenteeism and turnover.

Bank of America Stay Healthy Program

As part of the pilot program started in 1980, the Bank of America offered to pay the employee's share of the health insurance premium for one year if the bank had not paid any claims for that employee during the previous year. The bank monitored the claims experience of this group and a control group to study the program effects. The data in table 2.1 are from the first year of the program.

The data show that, not unexpectedly, incentives for lower utilization appear to affect lower utilizers only. The bank estimates that approximately $5,900 was saved through lower benefit payments. However, since most employees who did not file claims would not have done so anyway, the cost of the incentive in foregone employee premium contributions was $68,000. The bank extended the program for a second year but has now discontinued it.

Bank of America in November of 1982 initiated a two-year pilot program in Fresno County with Blue Shield to test the Stay

TABLE 2.1 Distribution of total claims per subscriber

Amount of claims	PILOT GROUP Number	% of total	CONTROL GROUP Number	% of total
$ 0	225	43.6	142	31.4
1–250	209	21.1	147	32.5
251–500	57	11.0	53	11.5
501–1,000	41	8.0	35	7.7
1,001–5,000	65	12.6	59	13.1
5,001–10,000	15	2.9	13	2.9
10,000 and above	4	.8	4	.9
	616	100.0	453	100.0

Well–Health Incentive Plan program. The insurance plan has $100 and $250 deductibles for individuals and families, respectively, with 20 percent coinsurance on the major medical. The bank has set up three groups of 500 to 600 employees each. Employees in the first group have a medical expense account set aside for them with contributions of $300 for individuals and $500 for families. However, instead of the medical expense account being used to pay for cost-sharing, it is used to pay for benefits until it is exhausted. Any amount left in the account at the end of the year is returned to the individual. For example, a single employee with $200 in medical bills in one year would pay the first $100 out-of-pocket for the deductible and have $80 taken out of his account. At the end of the year, he would receive the remaining $220 in cash. The first group also receives educational material about self-care and health promotion.

The second group will receive the same educational material as the first group but not the financial incentives. The third group is a control and will not receive either.

Blue Cross of Oregon Wellchec Program

This medical expense account program was started in 1981 for employees of the Pilot Rock School and has since been extended to another large group and to employees of Blue Cross. Its major distinguishing feature is that, to be eligible for cash payments, the employee must not use more than a preset number of sick days and must agree to achieve certain goals—e.g., to exercise or lose weight—that are incorporated into a point scoring system and administered on an honor system basis.

TABLE 2.2   Mobil Oil contribution bonus payments family coverage

	1977	1978	1979	1980	1981	1982
Average annual bonus	$ 55	$ 95	$103	$154	$150	$ 85
Maximum annual bonus	$108	$156	$161	$255	$197	$106
% employees receiving bonus	94%	85%	94%	85%	93%	86%

Blue Cross/Blue Shield of Virginia
Cash and Days Off Rewards

Employees of Blue Cross and Blue Shield of Virginia can earn a day off from work in any of three ways: by having one of six procedures performed on an outpatient basis rather than in the hospital; by limiting hospital maternity stays to three days; or by not receiving benefit payments in one year that exceed $75 for a single employee, $113 for an employee with a minor dependent, or $225 for a family.

Additionally, employees have a group incentive to reduce costs. Blue Cross has estimated the total cost of employee health benefits at $1.9 million. If these costs are less than $1.9 million, the employees will share 50 percent of the savings.

Mobil Oil Contribution Bonus

Beginning in 1977, the Mobil Oil Corporation initiated a program that rewards employees as a group for low utilization. Mobil's employees are divided into nine experience units along geographical and corporate functional lines. At the start of each year, Mobil determines how much the company will contribute. If health plan costs are below the company's contribution plan costs for a given unit, the employees in that unit receive a bonus equal to the difference. If plan costs exceed the company's contribution, employees pay the difference through payroll deduction.

Employees in most, but not all, experience units have received bonus payments. Table 2.2 provides information about bonus payments to date.

The program has not been evaluated. However, between 1977 and 1983, per employee premiums increased at annual rates of 15 percent for single persons and 16 percent for families, making it questionable whether the bonus is affecting utilization patterns dramatically.

Cash Awards for Early Obstetrical
and Gynecological Discharges

Several Blue Cross/Blue Shield plans have established cash award programs to reduce the length of stay for obstetrical and gynecological admissions. Blue Cross of Massachusetts, in cooperation with Melrose-Wakefield Hospital, has a pilot program that awards $100 to a mother who is discharged within 24 hours of delivery. An additional $100 is deposited in her physician's patient care fund, which can be used by the physician for otherwise uncovered services. In conjunction with this program, a maternity day care plan is offered that provides nursing and homemaker services for early discharge mothers. Money is also credited to the patient care fund for hysterectomy patients who are discharged early according to set criteria.

The New Hampshire Blue Cross/Blue Shield plan has established a similar arrangement with hospitals in Concord and Manchester. Mothers who return home within one day receive a $50 payment plus visiting nurse and homemaker services.

Medical Audit Rewards

Some companies (e.g., Control Data Corporation, General Mills) will share the savings that result when an employee finds an error on a hospital bill, e.g., charges for services not performed. General Mills shares 50 percent of the savings, and Control Data shares the full savings up to $100.

CHANNELING

Most benefits managers are well aware of the need for employees to understand their benefits and how to use them. Some, however, have found good communication materials alone to be insufficient and have initiated active programs to channel patients to particular providers based on cost and quality considerations. The recommended providers are generally not conceived of as constituting a preferred provider organization (see chapter 3). However, the logical next step is to formalize the process by having a list of providers judged to be efficient and to adopt plan design features that reward patients who use these providers. Doing so would, in effect, create a preferred provider arrangement.

One of the first such programs is the "medical information service" initiated in 1979 by Government Products Division of Pratt and

Whitney for its more than 8,000 employees in West Palm Beach, Florida. The initial thrust was to make fee information available, particularly for physician services. Program staff also offered individual counseling to employees and, over time, developed a reasonable knowledge of physician practice patterns and of which physicians were courteous and of high quality. They also promoted second opinions for surgery. Employees who used the service were expected to complete a form within 30 days providing feedback to the company. Company officials estimate that, over a two and a half year period, the program saved $175,000 for the company and $75,000 for employees, largely from steering patients to less expensive providers. A similar program has been implemented more recently for some 9,000 employees at Automatic Electric, a GTE subsidiary located outside of Chicago.

Together with Blue Cross/Blue Shield of Illinois, Zenith developed its "medical services advisory program," which was initiated in January 1983 for Zenith's 3,000 salaried employees in the Chicago area. Under this program, employees are required to talk to Zenith's medical advisor once they learn that they, or a member of their family, are scheduled for admission to a hospital. However, any change in treatment plan is totally voluntary. Employees are asked to provide the medical advisor with information regarding diagnosis, planned surgical procedures (if any), the hospital to be used, and the anticipated admission date, and length of stay. The medical advisor reviews whether hospitalization is necessary or, instead, whether the procedure could be performed on an ambulatory basis, and may also discuss with the employee the possible use of a less expensive facility, e.g., community rather than teaching hospital for routine surgery. Employees are encouraged to ensure that their physician understands that an overly long length of stay will result in avoidable cost-sharing expenses. If the employee desires, the medical advisor will discuss the case with the physician.

Although company policy mandates that all planned hospital admissions be reported, penalties have not as yet been instituted if the employee fails to do so, and the compliance rate has been roughly 50 percent. The company reports that the program has been popular with employees, who welcome assistance in dealing with the health care system. It hopes to negotiate the incorporation of a similar program into its union contracts.

Blue Cross/Blue Shield of Illinois is implementing similar approaches in other companies, including Illinois Tool Works, the clothing manufacturer Hartmax, and the publisher R. R. Donnelly.

In February 1983, Owens-Illinois initiated on a trial basis a "patient services program" for the company's 3,500 employees and dependents in Toledo, Ohio. It is staffed by two full-time nurses and one half-time nurse who are available to talk to employees and their dependents regarding preadmission testing, discharge planning, use of home health services, and so forth. The nurses also visit patients in the hospital, although some local area hospitals have resisted their presence. If the patient services program does not learn of an admission in advance, it is informed by the local professional review organization of the admission, and a nurse will visit the patient in the hospital to help with discharge planning. This service is voluntary with the patient; a retrospective review of the stay is performed for patients who refuse the service. If the program proves successful, the company, as a next step, plans to start recommending specific doctors and hospitals.

Another example is a system of service centers established by the teamsters union to service fourteen locals in various parts of New York, New Jersey, and Connecticut. Phone and walk-in advice is available on how to pick providers, and referrals to specific providers are given. The centers also provide information on second opinions for surgery, alcohol and drug abuse treatment, and various nonhealth matters, such as legal and financial. The centers also conduct hypertension control programs and health oriented workshops.

Finally, Coors Industries in Golden, Colorado, has established a referral program for mental health practitioners. This company has a self-insured and self-administered health benefits program that requires prior authorization of mental health benefits and also tries to match providers with the individual needs of employees.

CONCLUSION

Many companies view benefit package design as the linchpin of their cost-management strategy. As we have documented, changes are occurring, some in ways that would have been inconceivable a few years ago. Examples include mandatory or incentive second surgical opinion programs, the elimination of base programs with their first-dollar coverage, the rapid adoption of medical expense accounts, and efforts to channel patients to particular providers. Furthermore, employers who have changed their benefits have in many instances sought to increase the rationality of the system, e.g., by eliminating biases favoring inpatient care rather than, say, by restricting outpatient physician coverage or eliminating dental coverage.

Even more exciting is the willingness of some purchasers to manage their benefits actively, including explicitly attempting to change patient and purchaser behavior. As we have discussed, preadmission testing is an economy measure only if the tests are not re-peated once the patient is hospitalized. Similarly, home health benefits are more likely to result in savings if they are accompanied by an active discharge planning process that is managed or overseen by the purchaser rather than just the hospital. Some benefit programs are beginning to go even further and channel enrollees to specific providers.

Over the next few years, plan design will continue to be a dy-namic topic. First, the role of the carriers and third-party administra-tors will continue to change. Many purchasers have elected to self-administer out of frustration with the perceived lack of responsive-ness of carriers and third-party administrators. These carriers and third-party administrators, depending on one's perspective, have either been slow to adapt or are reflecting the demands of the major-ity of employers, who are still barely getting their feet wet in the complex world of cost containment. Inevitably, however, it is likely that their role must change and that they will become more forceful in tailoring benefits and in addressing delivery system issues. One question is whether these changes will be reflected in policies for small and medium sized groups, rather than only in the coverage of large groups. The majority of innovations to date have been designed by employers and negotiated with carriers. They are not reflected in the small group coverages for which the carrier is at risk.

One area deserving attention is that of plan complexity. The greatest communication program in the world cannot fully overcome the effect of a benefits structure that is inherently difficult to under-stand. For example, provisions allowing a carryover of unused de-ductible credits from one year to the next are often poorly understood. There may be a trade-off between simplicity and certain cost-containment objectives. A plan with numerous nonuniform coinsurance or deductible rates, however well-intentioned, can be confusing.

Another area that will receive increasing attention by insurers and employers relates to duplicate coverage, which is becoming in-creasingly widespread with the increase in two-earner families. One effect of duplicate coverage is to frustrate the cost-containment intent of good plan design, because the coverage under one policy typically fills in the cost-sharing in the second policy, thereby negating any in-tended restraining effect. An open issue is whether employers should develop standardized procedures that encourage two-earner families to have only a single policy. Individual companies have taken steps to address this matter, such as through increasing premium shares and, in a few instances, denying coverage altogether to dependents of heads of households. However, the topic deserves far more attention than it has received to date.

Finally, we believe that the next major step in benefit package design is for employers and other purchasers to be selective among, and negotiate with, providers. This will, of course, be most feasible in areas of high employment concentration or where several employers collaborate, through the mechanism of a coalition or otherwise. Perhaps the greatest potential for savings will come from channeling patients to specific providers judged to be cost effective. The data base for making these judgments is not easy to compile, particularly for physician services, but it can be done. In addition, purchasers will increasingly develop direct contracting arrangements, particularly with hospitals and pharmacies, and introduce plan design features to favor those providers and retail outlets that do enter into agreements.

All of this, of course, assumes a fundamental shift in philosophy in health benefits, i.e., from simply establishing the benefits package to managing the benefits. However critical plan design may be, a comprehensive strategy to manage health benefits entails a multiplicity of measures, reflecting individual circumstances, to be undertaken by the purchaser. This theme is articulated further in the concluding chapter of this book.

APPENDIX: PLAN CONTRACTING MECHANISMS

Many large purchasers (employers, union-management trust funds, multiemployer trusts, etc.) have changed contracting or funding mechanisms in recent years. Most noteworthy is the movement toward self-insurance, whereby the purchaser does not have insurance coverage as such and is fully at risk for the cost of health benefits. However, changes in contracting mechanisms do not by themselves impact on reimbursement or the delivery system, and the differences among them are less consequential than many people believe. Nonetheless, it is worth reviewing their origin and their implications, because they are not always well understood and are viewed by some as cost-containment measures by themselves.

Health insurance as we know it today originated during the depression when hospitals, facing large bad debts, joined together to form Blue Cross plans that would market coverage in order to assure themselves a source of income. Subsequently, Blue Shield plans were formed to reimburse physicians and other medical services. Most Blue Cross and Blue Shield plans are organized on a geographically franchised basis as nonprofit hospital or physician service corporations and are chartered under separate state legislation that is distinct from the insurance codes.

Commercial carriers first marketed health benefits aggressively after World War II. A major difference is in how they set their premiums. The Blue Cross plans community-rated their premiums; that is, they charged a single rate independent of the health risk of the individual enrolled. In contrast, commercial insurers began to relate premiums to enrollees' risk characteristics, such as their age, county of residence, sex, and occupational category. Ultimately, they began to experience-rate large groups: each individual group paid the carrier based on its own claims experience. Competitive pressures forced Blue Cross to follow suit or lose enrollment.

Today, most large groups are experience-rated. (The size at which groups should self-insure is a matter of judgment; as a general rule, 500 employees or family units is the bare minimum group size at which self-insurance should be contemplated.) Their premium payments to the carriers have two components. The first is retention, which covers the cost of administration—mostly claims processing—and profit. The purchaser typically agrees to pay a predetermined amount for retention or accepts a formula for calculating retention charges. The second component is the benefit payments. These are estimated prospectively. However, at the end of the year, any overestimate is returned to the purchaser as a dividend, and any underestimate is recaptured by increasing subsequent payments. (In practice, premiums are usually intentionally overestimated by some percentage, e.g., 5 percent, known as the margin, which assures that a dividend will result most of the time. If the margin is exceeded, the insurer can usually pass along the excess to the purchaser in subsequent years, unless the insured group switches carriers.) Even where there is not a retrospective adjustment based on actual experience, the prior year's experience is the major determinant of premium levels, and any over- or underestimates are typically built into the premiums in subsequent years.

Self-insurance essentially operates in the following manner. As with experience-rated insurance, the purchaser pays the claims-processing organization a prenegotiated amount to cover the cost of administration (unless the group, in addition to being self-insured, is also self-administered, as described below). The major difference is that, instead of paying premiums and receiving dividends at the end of the year that reflect actual experience, a separate account is established in the name of the employer out of which benefits are paid. The ultimate costs of benefits to the employer are roughly the same.

Self-insurance differs from experience rating in four significant respects. (1) The purchaser has a greater choice regarding the organization that processes claims. It can contract with insurance carriers; many large commercial companies report that more than one-third of their business is on a self-insured, or administrative services only (ASO), basis. It can contract with so-called third-party administrators, i.e., firms that are not licensed as insurance carriers but that specialize in processing claims under ASO agreements. Alternatively, it can administer the program itself, processing its own claims rather than using an outside contractor (this sometimes is referred to as self-managed). (2) Premiums of commercial insurers based in another state are subject to a state premium tax, typically 2 percent, whereas ASO contracts are not. Although the tax is technically on the insurer, it is passed along to the purchaser and reflected in premiums. (3) Under ERISA, self-insured plans are exempt from state insurance regulation. Although they are technically subject to federal regulation, the federal government has never shown any inclination to act. Thus, the purchaser can be relieved of minimum benefit package and other requirements (e.g., that mental health services be covered) by self-insuring. However, self-insuring purchasers conform as a matter of policy to the minimum benefit provisions of state law. (4) The purchaser maintains possession of financial reserves that are held to pay claims and thus earns investment income from them. However, investment income is often a subject of negotiation between the purchaser and the carrier for plans that do not self-insure.

Although these differences are meaningful, they do not in themselves have a direct impact on benefit payments, other than the exemption from state minimum benefit requirements. In any event, it is the purchaser, and not the carrier, that is at risk for large groups, and the carrier functions primarily as a claims processor and conduit of funds. Symbolically, however, the movement to self-insurance can be viewed as the one step that many purchasers understood and could take. It may also be a precursor to other, more forceful, actions. A frequently expressed complaint concerns the paucity of data that carriers generate. Some companies report that, by both switching to self-insurance and processing their own claims, they have enhanced their ability to generate data and conduct utilization review. In essence, these companies contend that carriers and third-party administrators have not been willing to address delivery system issues in as forceful a manner as they can do themselves.

In recent years, an additional form of contracting, referred to as minimum premium plans, has become increasingly common. Under a minimum premium plan, roughly 10 percent of the ultimate cost is paid as premiums, and the remaining 90 percent is in a self-insured account and is used to pay benefits. The major advantage of this approach over experience rating is that only the 10 percent paid in premiums is subject to the state premium tax, thereby effectively reducing the typical tax rate from 2 percent to 0.2 percent.

Available statistics on the prevalence of each contracting mechanism are only indicative, because there are no surveys based on scientifically designed random samples. The Hay-Huggins survey estimates that 10 percent of employers are self-insured and self-administered, 29 percent are self-insured with insurer or third-party administrator handling administration, 22 percent have a minimum premium arrangement, 35 percent are fully insured (mostly experience-rated), and 4 percent use a combination of arrangements. In contrast, in 1975, 83 percent of companies participating in the survey reported being fully insured.

REFERENCES

Finkel, M., H. Ruchlin, and S. Parsons. *Eight Years Experience with a Second Opinion Elective Surgery Program: Utilization and Economic Analyses.* Washington, D.C.: Department of Health and Human Services, Health Care Financing Administration, 1981.

Friedlob, A. "Medicare Second Surgical Opinion Programs: The Effect of Waiving Cost-Sharing." *Health Care Financing Review* 4(September 1982):99–106.

Galblum, T. "Second Surgical Opinions: What Have We Learned?" *Forum.* February 1980.

Health Care Cost Containment: A Second Biennial Survey—Participant Report. Walnut Creek, Calif.: Health Research Institute, 1981.

Joffe, J., and M. Schachter. "Program for Elective Surgical Second Opinion: Experience of Program Participants 1976–1977." New York: Blue Cross and Blue Shield of Greater New York, 1980. Mimeographed.

Long Term Care: Background and Future Directions. Washington, D.C.: Department of Health and Human Services, Health Care Financing Administration, 1981.

National HMO Census—1982. Excelsior, Minn.: InterStudy, 1983.

Newhouse, J.P., W.G. Manning, C.N. Morris, et al. "Some Interim Results from a Controlled Trial of Cost Sharing in Health Insurance." *New England Journal of Medicine* 305(January 1981): 1501–1507. (Also The Rand Corporation, R-2847-HHS, January 1982.)

1982 Survey of National Corporations on Health Care Cost Containment. Minneapolis: National Association of Employers on Health Care Alternatives, 1983.

Noncash Compensation Comparison. Philadelphia, Pa.: Hay-Huggins Co., 1983.

Orkand, D., F. Jagger, and E. Hurwitz. *Comparative Evaluation of Costs, Quality, and System Effects of Ambulatory Surgery Performed in Alternative Settings.* Silver Spring, Md.: Orkand Corp., 1977. (Contract with Health Care Financing Administration.)

Poggio, E.C., R. Kronick, H. Goldberg, and K. Calore. *Second Surgical Opinion Programs: An Investigation of Mandatory and Voluntary Alternatives.* Cambridge, Mass.: Abt Associates, Inc., 1981.

Roenigk, D., and L. Bartlett. *Controlling Medicaid Costs: Second Surgical Opinion Programs*. Washington, D.C.: National Governors' Association, 1982.

Strumpf, G.B. "Historical Evolution and the Political Process." In *Group and IPA HMOs*, edited by D.L. Mackie and D.K. Decker. Rockville, Md.: Aspen Publications, 1981.

Weissert, W.G. "Towards a Continuum of Care for the Elderly: A Note of Caution." *Public Policy* 29(Summer 1981): 331–40.

3

Alternative Health Care Delivery Systems: HMOs and PPOs

Jacob J. Spies, John Friedland, and Peter D. Fox

INTRODUCTION

One response to rising health care costs in recent years has been the evolution of health maintenance organizations (HMOs), which now represent roughly a $4 billion a year industry. More recently, preferred provider organizations (PPOs) have evolved as a vehicle for channeling patients to providers that are efficient or willing to give discounts.

This chapter discusses HMOs and PPOs. These two forms of alternative delivery systems differ widely in their respective stages of development and in the availability of relevant research. HMOs have become a mature industry and have been studied extensively. In contrast, PPOs are new; much less information about them is available, and little research has been completed. As a result, while the HMO discussion draws heavily on published sources (Luft 1981, various InterStudy publications) and on common wisdom, the information on PPOs comes mostly from interviews.

The remainder of this section defines HMOs and PPOs. The second section describes the basic models of each. The purchaser perspective is presented in the third section. The fourth outlines

TABLE 3.1   Numbers of HMOs and enrollment: 1974–83

	Number of plans	Growth rate	Enrollment (in millions)	Growth rate
June 1974	142		5.3	
June 1975	178	18.3%	5.7	7.5%
June 1976	175	−1.6	6.0	5.2
June 1977	165	−5.7	6.3	5.0
June 1978	198	20.0	7.3	15.8
June 1979	215	8.6	8.2	12.3
June 1980	236	9.8	9.1	10.9
June 1981	243	2.9	10.3	13.2
June 1982	265	9.1	10.8	4.8
June 1983	280	5.7	12.5	15.7

Source: InterStudy, National HMO Census (Excelsior, Minn., various years).

trends and future directions. The final section discusses the elements of viable HMOs and PPOs.

Although talking about different models of alternative delivery systems is instructive, these models blend into one another and form a continuum. Similarly, alternative delivery systems are arising that combine elements of different models.

Some 12.5 million Americans are enrolled in 280 HMOs, and roughly 40 percent of HMO members are in one of the nine Kaiser Plans (InterStudy 1983). As shown in table 3.1, this represents an increase of 70 percent in the number of plans and of 98 percent in enrollment over just a six-year period. HMOs assume a legal responsibility for financing and arranging to deliver a defined, comprehensive package of health care services. They receive premiums that are set in a competitive environment, thereby creating incentives to provide services efficiently and economically. If expenditures exceed revenues, the HMO is at risk for the loss, which is often shared with its participating doctors and/or hospitals.

As will be discussed in the next section, only a handful of PPOs are functioning, although several hundred are in various stages of planning, development, and initial marketing. The explosive level of interest and the newness of the phenomenon make it difficult to define a PPO or to estimate the magnitude of activity. As one observer aptly stated, "If you've seen one PPO, you've seen one PPO."* However, certain distinguishing characteristics are emerging.

*Max Fine, President of Max Fine Associates, quoted in Health Services Information, April 25, 1983, p. 1.

In a PPO, services are provided to enrollees by an organization or panel of providers (doctors, hospitals, dentists, etc.), usually at a discounted fee. The PPO can entail a single type of provider or a combination, e.g., both doctors and hospitals. Patients decide, service by service, whether to use participating providers. They are typically encouraged to do so through plan design features that significantly reduce or waive cost-sharing for services rendered by preferred providers.

There is no risk to the preferred providers, who charge agreed-upon fees. Any provider who no longer wishes to participate merely drops out. (Some alternative delivery systems that call themselves or are referred to as PPOs, such as the "Choice" plan of the Aetna Insurance Company, charge a premium and accept risk. We would consider these organizations to be prepaid health plans, or HMOs, rather than PPOs.) Providers usually agree to participate in a utilization review program. In addition to the potential for increased market shares, the incentives for providers to participate are guaranteed, rapid payment of claims (which improves cash flow and eliminates bad debts) and reduced paperwork because the plan is billed directly.

PPOs differ from HMOs in two principal respects. First, PPO patients, unlike HMO patients, are not restricted to using participating providers, although there are incentives for them to do so. Second, the financial risk is fully borne by the purchaser or carrier and not by the PPO.

One virtue of PPOs over HMOs is that they are easier and less expensive to form. There need not be an organization, per se, but only agreements with providers covering utilization controls, claim procedures, and payment arrangements. For this reason, some have adopted the term preferred provider arrangement instead of preferred provider organization.

In addition, PPOs are subject to less, if any, regulation. Because of the federal Employee Retirement Income Security Act of 1974 (ERISA), states are precluded from restricting the ability of self-insured groups, other than multiemployer trusts, to contract with PPOs. For insured groups, legislation does not seem to be necessary in most states, although several (Wisconsin, Michigan, Utah, Virginia, Connecticut, and California) have passed or are contemplating legislation to eliminate current provisions in state law that preclude carriers from selectively contracting with a limited number of providers.

The PPO is also potentially more attractive to employees, because they are not locked into a particular delivery system, and to providers, because of the absence of financial risk sharing.

BASIC MODELS

Health Maintenance Organizations

HMOs vary substantially in terms of how participating physicians are organized and paid. The two basic models are the prepaid group practice plan (PGPP) and the prepaid individual practice plan (PIPP). The two models, and the principal variant within each model, are described in this section. However, the distinctions are not rigid, and a number of plans are hybrids.

Prepaid Group Practice Plans (PGPPs)

PGPPs deliver the bulk of physician services to their enrollees at centralized ambulatory care centers staffed by multispecialty groups of participating doctors, who receive a significant portion of their income from salary. Physicians' incomes do not vary directly with the volume of services they provide to HMO enrollees. This organizational structure permits the plans to select participating doctors carefully, increases the opportunities for informal peer interaction and shared medical records, and provides a focused peer review to reinforce physician commitment to HMO objectives and procedures. These factors facilitate control of utilization and coordination of care. However, this control may be largely informal and exercised primarily through peer pressure.

The three HMO models within the PGPP category are known as staff, group, and network. In the staff model, participating physicians are salaried employees of the HMO who provide most outpatient services at the plan's multispecialty ambulatory care center(s). Only rarely do these physicians provide a significant volume of fee-for-service care, and any resulting income accrues to the HMO rather than the individual physician.

In contrast, group model HMOs arrange for physician services by contracting with an independent multispecialty group practice, whose members then become the plan's participating doctors. Commonly, the group practice predates the HMO, functioning on a fee-for-service basis in one or more ambulatory care centers. The HMO pays the group a negotiated capitation—a fixed sum per enrollee per month. Referrals to nonparticipating doctors are usually also paid out of the capitation. There may also be a bonus plan to create an incentive for doctors to control hospital costs.

Finally, network models closely resemble group model HMOs, except that the HMO contracts with two or more separate independent group practices. Each group receives capitation payments from the HMO for enrollees who designate that medical group. Most groups that are part of a network also continue to serve fee-for-service patients, and the clinical facilities are usually owned by the physicians rather than the HMO.

Prepaid Individual Practice Plans (PIPPs)

These are also known as individual practice associations (IPAs). Rather than relying upon centralized group practices, individual practice plans generally contract with solo practitioners and small, mostly single-specialty, groups. These HMOs commonly have large panels of participating physicians. Consumers are often attracted by easier access to primary care sites and the wider choice of physicians, which may include their present doctors, than is the case for PGPPs.

Most PIPPs reimburse participating physicians on a fee-for-service basis. Fee schedules, or maximum fee levels, are established. When claims are processed, the fees are typically reduced below the scheduled amount to protect against the possibility that total physician payments might exceed the budget for physician services. The fee reductions are accumulated in individual physician accounts and are paid back at the end of the year if budget targets are met. In addition, any surplus in the plan's budget for physician services may be distributed, usually in proportion to the volume of services rendered, if it is not needed to meet cost overruns in other areas, such as hospitalization. Also, as in the PGPP models, participating doctors may receive bonuses if hospital costs are below plan projections. Thus, the financial risks and incentives operate to encourage cost-effective practice patterns. However, because the physician is compensated in proportion to total services rendered, the incentives are collective rather than individual, thus often necessitating more extensive utilization controls than in the PGPP model.

A few PIPPs, such as Maryland IPA and HMO of Pennsylvania, use a different approach, called the primary care network model, for reimbursing their participating primary care physicians. In these plans, an enrollee's access to nonemergency covered services is controlled by a single primary care physician, who receives a per enrollee capitation payment. The payment amount may vary with the age and sex of the enrollee but does not vary with the volume of services that the primary physician provides. A second capitation-based account is established for each primary care doctor and is used to pay for referral services ordered by that physician. At the end of the year the doctor receives a share of any surplus in this account but must pay back part of any deficit. Thus, unlike other HMO models, the financial risk of each primary care doctor is dependent solely upon the expenses generated by his or her own panel of enrollees. Hospital costs may or may not be included in the referral capitation.

Mixed models

A number of plans incorporate elements from more than one of the models discussed above. For example, some PIPPs, such as North Central Health Protection Plan in Wisconsin, utilize multispecialty group practices in addition to solo or single-specialty groups. Furthermore, the group practice physicians may be salaried employees of the HMO, in a separately capitated medical group, or paid on a modified fee-for-service basis. Some staff and group model plans include only the primary care specialties in their group practices and contract for specialty services on a per session or fee-for-service basis. For example, Medical South in Boston, a staff model HMO, refers out most specialty care. Finally, network and group model plans may use salaried physicians to staff some of their ambulatory care centers or to fill certain slots in their physician staffing arrangements.

Preferred Provider Organizations

A distinction should be made between PPOs that are operational—meaning that they have some enrollment, however minimal —and those that are in various stages of planning, development, or initial marketing operational. The former are few in number, perhaps around 20. In contrast, the latter category represents a large number, amounting to several hundred.

It is also important to realize that the concept of enrollment differs between an HMO and a PPO, since PPO "enrollees" can use any provider. Enrollment simply means that there is a preferred provider agreement with a third-party payer or purchaser that allows the enrollee to use the PPO, not that he/she necessarily does so. A common reason that enrollees do not use preferred providers is that these providers may not be conveniently located. Another reason could be that a specific service or specialty might not be available. Furthermore, an employer or other group can enter into agreements with several PPOs, resulting in individuals being enrolled in more than one PPO.

Operational PPOs

Several PPOs were initiated in the late 1970's, before the term was coined. The biggest concentration is in Denver, where PPO activity was largely stimulated by a single person, Samuel Jenkins, vice-president of the Martin E. Segal Co., a benefits consulting firm with a large self-insuring trust fund clientele. (For more information on PPOs in Denver, see Fox and Tell 1983.)

Starting in the early 1970s, Jenkins negotiated preferred provider agreements with Denver hospitals that were heavily used by his clients and that he believed to be efficient. Discounts, generally between 6 and 15 percent, were agreed to. Subsequently, preferred provider agreements were developed for dental and eye care.

In 1978, the first physician PPO was formed with fee-for-service doctors in independent practices who had admitting privileges at St. Anthony's Hospital. It is the physician PPOs that have received national attention. Subsequently, five other physician PPOs were established, each with membership open to the physicians who were associated with individual hospitals and who elected to participate. They are: the Organization of Independent Physicians, physicians associated with St. Joseph's Hospital; Mountain Medical Affiliates, physicians associated with the three component hospitals of Presbyterian–St. Luke's Medical Center; Front Range Medical Center, comprised of osteopathic doctors associated with Valley View Hospital, part of the Humana chain; Rocky Mountain Medical Group, doctors associated with Rocky Mountain Osteopathic Hospital; and Chevy Creek Associated Physicians, affiliated with Rose Medical Center.

At present, the PPOs have contracts with trust funds only, mostly clients of the Martin E. Segal Co., although one PPO says that it is in the process of negotiating contracts with two firms. At least 70,000 employees plus their dependents are in trust funds with one or more such contracts.

The administrative mechanism for each PPO is fairly modest. In some cases there is only a part-time administrator. Plan marketing and the education of union members regarding the PPO are conducted by the Martin E. Segal Co. and representatives of the various union trusts. Claims review and processing are handled by third-party administrators—firms that specialize in processing claims for self-insured groups.

Physician reimbursement is based on fee schedules or maximum allowances, which each PPO has independently developed. These allowances average about 20 percent below average charges in the community. Except for a modest copayment (five dollars per visit) on office visits that is collected directly from the patient, participating physicians agree to accept the maximum allowances as payment in full. One PPO has recently begun to require that physician members cannot belong to another PPO and that they must admit to the PPO hospital if there is no medical contraindication. None of the Denver PPOs has established criteria for selecting physicians based upon practice patterns, and thus there is no reason to believe that they are either more or less efficient than other physicians in the community.

Med Network was organized in 1977 by Ad Mar Corporation, a third-party administrator headquartered in Santa Ana, California. Ad Mar dealt initially with physicians since, at that time, the hospitals were not interested in PPO agreements. The objective was to organize a plan that would compete with the HMOs and have a measurable impact on health costs. Physicians agreed to fee reductions (up to 20 percent depending on existing profiles) and a strong utilization management program, including admission controls. Starting around 1979, a plan was marketed that included reduced cost-sharing for patients who used preferred providers. There are now 40–50 hospitals participating and 6,000 physicians. Currently, the PPO has contracts with roughly 120 groups, representing some 80,000 employees and dependents.

Humana, Inc., a for-profit hospital firm headquartered in Louisville, Kentucky, has pilot programs in operation in Jackson, Mississippi, and Fort Lauderdale, Florida. These are hospital-based PPOs with physicians recruited from the hospitals' medical staffs. Both hospitals and physicians discount charges by about 15 percent. Practice patterns were not examined in selecting physicians. However, Humana representatives say that they might do so once they have sufficient data. As of the fall of the 1983, the PPO in Jackson had 7,000 potential users and the Fort Lauderdale PPO had 28,000.

Effective January 1, 1981, the American Family Corporation, an insurance firm in Columbus, Georgia, offered its employees a PPO as an alternative within the company-sponsored group program. The PPO was developed by a subsidiary of the company, Medical Cost Management System, and is not currently being marketed to other companies. Participating physicians agree to accept 90 percent of their usual fees as full payment, with the exception of surgery. If surgery is performed in a hospital on an outpatient basis, the physician is paid 100 percent of his fee. If the same procedure is performed in the physician's office, he or she is paid 125 percent of his fee. Physicians are selected personally by the company's medical director on the basis of credentials and known practice habits. Some 102 physicians are currently participating, representing about 60 percent of community physicians. Employees who use participating physicians are reimbursed in full. Those who use nonparticipating physicians face 20 percent coinsurance. The company reports having realized savings under this plan. The average cost of a hospital admission for nonparticipating physicians in 1982 was $2,614.48 compared to $1,809.45 for participating physicians.

Universal Health Network was established in 1981 by the Lutheran Hospital Society of Southern California, a nonprofit multi-hospital system, for its own 5,000 employees, using the hospitals in the system and the 1,300 doctors with admitting privileges. The PPO originally was not selective. However, it is improving its utilization review capacity and identifying any inefficient providers. An employee who uses a member provider does not face cost-sharing, whereas one who does not faces 20 percent coinsurance. Universal Health Network has not marketed outside the hospital system but is considering doing so.

PPOs under development

Because of the fast rate at which PPOs are forming, the uncertainties regarding the seriousness of intent of some efforts, and the presence of groups that perhaps inappropriately label themselves as PPOs, the numbers of PPOs that are being formed cannot be known with any degree of certainty. The American Hospital Association estimates that 611 hospitals are interested in PPOs, and most states have between five and ten in some stage of development—some states (e.g., California) more than ten. Thus, there are clearly several hundred in various stages of discussion or development.

Most of the emerging PPOs are being initiated by one of three groups: (1) providers, (2) carriers and third-party administrators, and (3) purchasers. Other PPOs are being initiated by individual consultants and entrepreneurs. The following discussion of the three major categories is not an attempt to classify PPO development rigidly. Indeed, the potential success of PPOs may well lie in their flexibility and ability to respond to specific organizational and community needs.

Provider-originated model. Provider-originated PPOs (both hospital and physician) are usually formed to capture or maintain a share of the market and to compete with other delivery mechanisms, primarily HMOs. Hospitals generally build the physician component of the PPO around their own medical staff, i.e., those fee-for-service physicians that have admitting privileges. They also usually use their existing utilization review or medical audit committee structure to monitor utilization.

Physician organizations are also forming PPOs as a strategy for protecting or increasing their share of the market. While most of these groups have a common hospital relationship, some do not. As with hospitals, physician groups tend to rely primarily on discounted fees to obtain a competitive advantage.

Unlike HMOs, provider-based PPOs can accommodate virtually any benefit package. They offer a delivery mechanism for the use of a third party, such as a corporation, an employer, a trust fund, or an insurance company. Most provider-originated PPOs are not able to document that they are efficient. However, one likely possibility is that some lower cost providers will form PPOs and market their practice patterns rather than discounts. For example, suburban hospitals in Cleveland have developed PPOs to compete with the more expensive downtown hospitals.

Three examples of provider originated PPOs in the formative stage can be found in San Diego, where the medical staff of Scripps Memorial Hospital has formed a separate corporation that constitutes a PPO. Services will be marketed to industry and insurance companies by the hospital through a joint venture between hospital and the medical group. The Scripps Clinic and Foundation, not part of Scripps Memorial Hospital, though also in San Diego, is developing two PPOs. One will serve the local market and the other, in conjunction with other large California clinics (e.g., Palo Alto, Riverside, Santa Barbara), will provide services through a statewide network. The latter plan divides the state into ten regions and designates a clinic as responsible for a particular region.

National Medical Enterprises and Hospital Corporation of America, both large for-profit hospital chains, are developing PPOs in California and Florida, respectively. The Franklin County Public Hospital in Greenfield, Massachusetts, is forming a plan exclusively to serve the local TRW plant. Five low-cost hospitals in Milwaukee and their medical staffs are developing a PPO that does not entail fee discounts as such. A strong program to review utilization and fees is contemplated in order to keep costs competitive.

Purchaser-originated model. Industry is beginning to form, or encourage the formation of, PPOs. Some corporations and coalitions of companies are identifying physicians and hospitals they consider cost-effective, with the intent of providing an incentive to employees through benefit plan design to encourage the use of those providers. With few exceptions, industry appears to be interested in efficient practice patterns, not just discounted fees. The industry-initiated cost-management model PPO can be administered directly by a company that is self-insured or by an insurance carrier or third-party administrator.

Most of the purchaser or purchaser-provider coalitions are examining the opportunities offered by PPOs; the U.S. Chamber of Commerce Clearinghouse on Coalitions estimates the figure at perhaps 75 percent. Some, such as the San Diego Coalition, were encouraged by the Robert Wood Johnson Affordable Health Care Grant Program. A planning grant has been awarded to that coalition to develop a communitywide PPO to serve member firms, which represent 60 percent of employees in the Greater San Diego area. The primary criterion in the provider selection process is low utilization rather than the willingness to discount fees. This PPO, the Community Care Network (CCN), is targeted for operation in August 1984.

A large number of major corporations are seriously evaluating the possibility of a PPO for at least one location. Examples are Rohr Industries and Cubic Industries in San Diego; Digital Equipment, Bank of Boston, and Norton Manufacturing in Massachusetts; and ALCOA, DuPont, CitiCorp, Ford, Hewlett-Packard, General Motors, General Electric, Stouffers, and United Technologies.

Third-party-originated model. This category includes PPOs being developed by the Blues, insurance companies, third-party administrators, PIPPs, and foundations for medical care (FMCs). PIPPs may be in the best position of any sponsoring party to identify providers (both physicians and hospitals) that can be considered truly cost-effective, because of the data systems they must develop to conduct utilization review. PIPPs and FMCs that are developing PPOs include: Greater San Diego Health Plan, Physicians Health Plan (Minneapolis), Tufts Associated Health Plan (Boston), Greater San Diego FMC, and San Joaquin FMC. The PPO may be either a general offering to their customers or a response to a specific request from a single large client. These plans are generally built around a fee discount but may take practice patterns into consideration. However, one open issue is whether carriers are in a position to select among providers or take other measures that run the risk of antagonizing portions of the provider community.

Third-party administrators are forming PPOs as a service to their self-insured clients. Ad Mar and the Martin E. Segal Co. were among the first, as described earlier, and U.S. Administrators is considering forming a PPO-type program in northern California.

Many Blue Shield and Blue Cross plans are actively developing PPOs. For example, Virginia Blue Cross sought a Robert Wood Johnson grant to develop a communitywide PPO. Blue Cross of Southern California has been active in PPO development, especially in the San Diego area in cooperation with Cubic Industries. The "Aware" plan developed by Minnesota Blue Cross has attracted more hospital members than Blue Cross anticipated.

The commercial insurance industry has embraced PPOs much more rapidly than it did HMOs. While it took years to accept the term HMO (many companies still have trouble), the Health Insurance Association of America (HIAA) established a PPO subcommittee quite early. HIAA, and most major commercial carriers, are examining the PPO concept as a health management device for its group health policyholders and as a marketing tool for attracting new business. Most companies are reluctant to discuss specific plans at this time. However, the following are some examples: Mutual of Omaha is developing a nationwide PPO in cooperation with the Medical Group Management Association and the American Group Practice Association; Prudential is developing a plan in Massachusetts; and John Hancock Mutual Life is developing a PPO that will likely include an enrollment requirement intended to give consumers the perception of being committed to using participating providers.

PURCHASER PERSPECTIVES

This section discusses some of the positive and negative aspects of HMOs and PPOs from the perspective of major purchasers, particularly employers.

Reasons for Supporting HMOs and PPOs

Increasing insurance costs

Health insurance premiums have skyrocketed. Between 1979 and 1981 the private health insurance industry's aggregate premiums rose from $56 billion to $73 billion, a 30 percent increase in two years (Carroll and Arnett 1981). Faced with an increasingly unacceptable health insurance burden, employers are exploring alternative delivery systems that may be able to reduce costs.

Increasing presence of "brand name" HMOs

Employers are concerned about the possible administrative, financial, and morale problems should their employees enroll in an HMO that denies needed services, provides poor quality of care, or fails. The involvement of sponsors having extensive prior HMO experience, a known commitment to the HMO concept, and access to large financial sums is, therefore, quite comforting.

Some large and well-respected HMOs operate only in a single city. However, an important and growing segment of the industry consists of the national HMO firms, so called by InterStudy, a Minneapolis-based research organization known for its work on HMOs. The 10 such firms include 63 HMOs and account for roughly 51 percent of total national enrollment (Shadle 1983). Among the organizations that are considered national firms are the Kaiser Foundation Health Plans, Prudential Insurance (PruCare), CIGNA Corp. (INA Healthplans), John Hancock (Hancock-Dikewood), Charter Med, Healthplans Corp., and Maxicare. Another company moving into this arena is Co-Med of Columbus, Ohio. Surveys by InterStudy, Ernst and Whinney, and the Congressional Research Service indicate that many of these experienced, capable, and well-capitalized organizations are planning to form or acquire HMOs. Blue Cross HMOs, too, benefit from high brand recognition, although most of their 54 HMOs, which account for another 10 percent of total enrollment, operate independently of one another. As discussed in the next section, PPO chains are likely to evolve, and these too will be attractive to employers because they will allow access to a geographically dispersed provider base through a single contract.

The established track record

Usually, innovations are immediately adopted by only a small portion of people or businesses; many more assume a wait-and-see attitude. Over time, observation of the innovation combined with positive accounts from early adopters overcome earlier concerns. HMOs have been established in half of all standard metropolitan statistical areas (SMSAs). However, in just under half of these SMSAs, the first HMO was established after 1974. In many areas with HMOs, enrollment is still under 3 percent of the population, whereas it is as high as 20 percent or 30 percent in other areas where prepaid plans have longer histories. In contrast, employers are not approaching PPOs with the same level of suspicion, although many are adopting wait-and-see attitudes.

Reliance on private financing

Federal grants and loans, which financed a considerable portion of HMO development during the 1970s, created discomfort for many in the business community who favored private rather than public sector approaches. Some employers were also influenced by complaints emanating from the medical community that public subsidies of HMOs constituted unfair competition. With the phasing out of federal grants and loans, these philosophical objections will diminish. Because of the low start-up and operational costs, availability of financing is much less of an issue for PPOs.

Provider acceptance

Although the majority (60 percent) of non-HMO physicians still express unfavorable attitudes towards HMOs (Louis Harris and Associates 1982), there are indications that provider acceptance is increasing. Physicians in multispecialty group practices have increased from 7.6 percent (24,000) of active physicians in 1969 to 12.0 percent (54,000) in 1980 (*American Medical News* 1982). The number of groups (multispecialty and others) reporting participation in prepaid plans increased from 396 to 1,884 during this same period.

The increasing supply of physicians and the high cost of establishing a practice are making HMOs a more attractive practice option. Physicians who report being more familiar than the average with the HMO concept are more likely to have a favorable attitude toward HMOs, and the attitudes of physician in residency training programs are more favorable than those of other physicians (Louis Harris and Associates 1982). This same Louis Harris survey reported that 57 percent of physicians believe that HMOs contain costs; a similar survey in 1978 reported a figure of only 28 percent (1978 data reported in Bryant and Boscarino 1979).

As physicians and hospitals increasingly participate in HMOs, these plans are less prone to be characterized as unacceptable or unethical. This diminished controversy reduces the reluctance of business to deal with them. In contrast to the early days of HMOs, many physicians appear eager to join PPOs. Thus physician opposition is unlikely to be an issue from the perspective of most employers.

Concerns with HMOs and PPOs

Selection issues

Many employers fear that healthier and younger employees choose (or would choose) to enroll in HMOs, leaving a higher cost segment of their work force in the conventional insurance plan. Since the conventional plan is typically experience-rated and the HMO is community-rated, employer expenditures rise if the conventional plan has a disproportionate number of high cost enrollees. Because payments to the PPO are simply reflected in the experience of the conventional plan, this issue does not arise for PPOs.

Doubts regarding whether employers share in savings

Many employers are comfortable in offering HMOs because they are attractive to employees, and do not view them as a vehicle for reducing the costs of health benefits. Others seek to achieve immediate or long-term savings. One way that savings are achieved is through the HMOs' introducing a market discipline that changes the behavior of fee-for-service providers as a competitive response. However, evidence is lacking that HMOs induce other providers and insurers to become more efficient. In fact, some employers contend that offering a HMO may weaken their bargaining position with their regular carrier and lead to increased premiums. Recent polls of employers, nationally and in Massachusetts, reflect doubt among employers that HMOs do reduce total costs. Employers clearly achieve savings when the HMO premium is lower than the employer's contribution to the conventional plan. This typically arises only when the employer offers comprehensive paid-in-full benefits.

Administrative burden

A substantial minority of employers are concerned about the administrative costs of setting up and maintaining multiple choice of health plans. Among the burdens cited are multiple contract negotiations, differential payroll deductions, additional paperwork, frustration at HMOs' limited ability to tailor benefit packages, and additional demands upon personnel staff for explanations of program options. A recent example of negative reaction among employers was the opposition of the business community to proposals to require that employers offer all federally qualified HMOs. One advantage of the PPO is that the administrative burden is less, because a formal enrollment process is not required.

Employer exposure, HMO stability, and quality of care

There have been well-publicized, if isolated, instances of employees facing bills for services rendered by HMOs that subsequently went bankrupt. The employees often turn to their employer who, by offering the HMO, is viewed as having, at least tacitly, endorsed it. In addition, concerns about being blamed by employees dissatisfied with the HMO's quality or style of care deter other employers from being more supportive. Whether employers will perceive themselves, or be perceived as, responsible for the quality of care of PPO providers is an open issue.

Limited service area

HMOs have limited service areas, but Americans are highly mobile. Employers express concern about service availability in cases where an employee is outside of the service area, as well as the portability of benefits when an employee is transferred to another location. The PPO obviously would be limited to the service area of the providers, although many are based on networks of providers that cover a broad geographic area. A concern of many employers is that a PPO contract entails offering a benefit that is, in practice, not available to all employees.

TRENDS AND FUTURE DIRECTIONS

Past attempts to predict HMO growth have been far afield of the actual occurrences. While we hope that our forecasts will be closer to the mark, it should be recognized that the future will reflect the interplay of a multiplicity of factors.

Growth

The number of HMOs will continue to increase throughout this decade, although perhaps at a slower rate. The slower growth will result from the consolidations or closings of smaller plans already operating as well as fewer new starts. Although new investment capital will be attracted to the HMO field, it will go largely to the most promising and well managed plans. Little will be available for marginal plans, and the number of consolidations and failures will increase as a weeding-out process occurs over the next several years.

Although enrollment gains in mature HMO markets will moderate as saturation is approached, growth should accelerate in other markets as a result of increasing public familiarity with the HMO concept, better name recognition as HMO chains expand, greater cost-sharing in many conventional insurance plans, and the development of Medicare and Medicaid policies that are supportive of alternative delivery systems.

The development of PPOs may reduce enrollment growth somewhat. However, a projected annual growth of around 10 percent seems reasonable, resulting in 30 million HMO enrollees by 1990.

PPO growth is less predictable. The greatest unknown is their ability to gain acceptance by large purchasers, which in turn depends on their demonstrating that they represent efficient delivery mechanisms. We expect that many of the PPOs in the discussion or forma-

TABLE 3.2   Enrollment and plan growth by type of plan
1978–82

Number of plans/enrollment	August 1978	June 1982	Percent increase
NUMBER			
All plans	203	265	30.5%
Prepaid group practices	137	168	22.6
Staff	54	57	5.6
Group	76	80	5.3
Network	7	31	342.9
Prepaid individual practice plans	66	97	47.0
ENROLLMENT (in thousands)			
All plans	7,471	10,831	45.0%
Prepaid group practices	6,679	9,361	40.2
Staff	961	1,618	68.4
Group	4,670	5,970	27.8
Network	1,048	1,773	69.2
Prepaid individual practice plan	793	1,471	85.5

Sources: U.S. Dept. of Health, Education, and Welfare, Office of HMOs, *National HMO Census of Prepaid Plans, 1978* (Washington, D.C.: GPO, n.d.).

InterStudy, *National HMO Census — 1982* (Excelsior, Minn., 1983).

tion stage will have difficulty obtaining contracts with third-party payers and, thus, will cease to exist.

By the same token, a number of large companies are engaged in efforts to identify efficient providers in areas of high employment concentration. It seems likely that many of these companies will create incentives through plan design or other mechanisms to use certain providers and disincentives to using inefficient providers. The disincentives, in addition to higher cost-sharing, could include prior authorization or even the outright refusal to reimburse selected providers. However structured, these incentives and disincentives create a preferred provider structure.

Plan Structure

As shown in table 3.2, both the number of plans and enrollment have increased significantly in recent years. However, the enrollment growth among staff and group models has come primarily from existing plans rather than from new plans. PIPPs have had enormous growth in both. However, the number of PIPPs peaked at 97, the same number as in 1982, and between 1980 and 1982, enrollment declined 13 percent, from 1,694,000 to 1,471,000.

New HMO starts by the existing national HMO chains have been predominantly, though not exclusively, of the PGPP type. A variety of factors contribute to this preference. The evidence on cost control is more convincing for PGPPs, and the process of developing PGPPs may be subject to more standardization, being a closed system to a greater extent than PIPPs. The identification of existing, cost-efficient multispecialty group practices is a relatively simple process for the national HMO firms, especially those that are affiliated insurance carriers and have extensive data on practice patterns. Also, PIPPs often face significant operational management problems, stemming from the need to coordinate a large panel of physicians (and, commonly, other providers) having weaker ties to the HMO. This characteristic accounts for financial failures being more common among PIPPs than PGPPs.

If these trends continue, and if new starts by the HMO chains become a larger component of total new starts as projected, PGPPs (already representing two of every three HMO plans) will be ever more dominant among HMOs.

It is also likely that some PIPPs will use their provider base to develop a PPO as an additional line of business to their prepaid health plan. Physician Health Plan in Minneapolis has already begun writing group contracts that permit enrollees to use any provider but with substantial deductibles and copayments when nonparticipating providers are used.

Affiliations between existing HMOs will not be limited to smaller plans in danger of failing. Larger independent plans, faced with growing competition from the expanding chains, will seek out one another to achieve greater administrative flexibility. These plans will position themselves to protect their markets from erosion by pooling managerial talent, sharing utilization and underwriting data, achieving administrative economies of scale (such as through centralized discount purchasing or standardized information and control systems), or possibly merging to form their own chains. Four major PGPPs from coast to coast have already joined together to study the feasibility of joint ventures, including the possible formation of for-profit corporations.

The structures of PPOs will continue to evolve and diversify. PPO networks, both national and statewide, are already developing.

TABLE 3.3   HMO sponsors

Type of sponsor	# HMOs pre-1970	# HMOs in 1982	% Sponsors pre-1970	% Sponsors in 1982
Consumer/community	15	72	35.7	22.2
Group practices	5	55	11.9	17.0
"Blues"	1	51	2.4	15.7
Hospital	1	44	2.4	13.6
Commercial carrier	2	32	4.7	9.9
Medical society/ other physicians	4	40	9.5	12.3
University	3	12	7.1	3.7
Corporation	4	10	9.5	3.1
Labor	7	8	16.7	2.5
	42	324	99.9	100.0

Sources: Robert Shouldice and Katherine Shouldice, *Medical Group Practice and Health Maintenance Organizations* (Washington, D.C.: Information Press, 1978), chapter 2.

National Association of Employers for Health Care Alternatives, *National Directory of HMOs*, first and second editions. (Minneapolis).

Group Health Association of America, *National HMO Census Survey, 1977* (Washington, D.C., n.d.).

U.S. Department of Health, Education and Welfare, Office of HMOs, *National HMO Census of Prepaid Plans 1978* (Washington, D.C.: GPO, n.d.).

InterStudy, *Hospital Sponsored HMOs, 1982* (Excelsior, Minn., July 1982), 3.

Notes: This table reflects only HMOs with known sponsors. Some HMOs with more than one sponsor are counted more than once.

Sponsorship

The last decade has witnessed dramatic shifts in HMO sponsorship, as shown in table 3.3. This table compares the sponsorship for HMOs formed through 1970 with that of HMOs in existence in 1982. The percent classified as consumer or community based dropped from 36 percent to 22 percent, and the percent that were sponsored by labor unions decreased from 17 percent to 2.5 percent. The most dramatic increases among the categories that represent a substantial presence were by carriers (both commercial and the Blues), hospitals, and group practices.

One issue for the future is the impact of the phaseout of the federal subsidies authorized by the HMO Assistance Act of 1973 combined with the awakening by health care providers and third-party payers to the significant impact that HMOs can have on their businesses and practices. Between 1974 and 1981 more than 300 organizations had received $330 million of federal financial assistance. Private investors accounted for approximately an additional $1.1 billion (65 percent invested by Kaiser). However, federal assistance has been discontinued, which creates an ever greater demand for private capital. The Congressional Budget Office has estimated that during the 1980s $225 million will need to be invested in HMOs for every one million new enrollees.

With public financing diminishing, the industry must turn to the private sector for support. HMOs have appeal as investments because of their ability to deliver comprehensive benefits at lower cost than indemnity plans and because of the very attractive return on equity demonstrated by successful HMOs, as well as the growth potential of good young plans in this relatively new industry; there is a growing number of sophisticated investors active in the field.

The trend toward HMO affiliations (chains) will continue in response to both marketing and financing factors, mirroring the growth in affiliations over the last few years among both for-profit and non-profit hospitals. With the turn to private financing, the incentives to reduce start-up costs (both pre- and postoperational) will increase, and parties with prior HMO experience and experienced HMO managers will be best able to accomplish this objective. Employer and employee market acceptance will also be facilitated by name identification. The constraint on affiliating is much more likely to be the limited interest of chains in signing up new affiliates than plan disinterest in such affiliations. HMOs that are most attractive for takeover will have one or more assets (facilities, physician organization, employer or union relationships, market position) that the chain finds politically or financially compelling or will be in markets in which the chain, for competitive reasons, especially values rapid entry. Thus, new starts by these HMO chains will likely be concentrated among the most attractive, identifiable market opportunities. To date, these seem to be primarily in rapidly growing communities of one-half million or more that are not yet served by a well-established HMO.

The major chains will continue to be operated mostly by for-profit companies and private insurance companies, with the exception of Kaiser-Permanente. PPO chains will also be developed by private insurance companies, third-party administrators and the Blues—primarily for national account clients. Efforts of Mutual of Omaha are an example.

To date, only a handful of plans have converted from not-for-profit to for-profit status. Conversions and for-profit start-ups will accelerate as plans increasingly compete with one another for access to capital.

Providers (hospitals and physicians) will be the primary non-chain sponsors, but their level of HMO involvement is likely to be diluted by their growing interest in PPOs. The extent of this effort will depend upon the yet unknown ability of PPOs to become an important market force.

Antitrust Considerations

The applicability of antitrust laws to the health field is complicated and is particularly uncertain for PPOs. The following are some of the major considerations in determining whether or not a PPO is in violation.

Who are the controlling decision makers in the PPO? There is less likely to be an antitrust issue if the carrier or purchaser controls the PPO than if providers do so.

If providers do control the PPO, what roles do they play in decision making? For example, if the PPO is provider-controlled, the likelihood of an antitrust violation is lessened if it markets only its utilization review capacity, leaving the negotiation of payment levels to the individual purchasers or carriers and providers.

If the response to either of these questions is favorable, then the likelihood of an antitrust violation is small. If not, two other factors become important. Is the PPO offering a new product or service? The PPO has a stronger antitrust defense if it is offering a new product than if it is not. For example, even though a PIPP-type of HMO sets rates, the fact that prepayment is a new product distinct from traditional fee-for-service medicine is a strong defense. Thus, the courts may be asked to pass judgment on whether PPOs are, in fact, a new way of organizing or paying for medical care.

What share of the local market does the PPO represent? Even if all of the above considerations suggest the possibility of an antitrust violation, the courts might well rule in favor of the PPO if, in any market area, its participants do not represent a substantial share of services delivered by any provider class (e.g., physicians, hospitals, dentists).

Operational Trends

The same pressure that led the Blues to abandon community rating and adopt experience rating will also affect HMOs, although perhaps not to the same degree. One of the stresses some HMOs will face involves deciding whether to retain federal qualification or, instead, respond to the demands of the marketplace for experience rating. Federal qualification requires community rating (or community rating by class) but also can improve access to employment-based groups.

These same competitive pressures will also force PIPPs to become more selective about whom they allow as participating physicians. Those who prefer more elaborate, intensive styles of medicine will be increasingly discouraged from participating. Other measures will also be taken by these plans to control costs, including concentrating admissions in lower priced and/or more efficient hospitals.

To supplement premium revenues and make better use of participating professionals and facilities, HMOs will develop new lines of business. PPO plans have already been mentioned as one area into which some HMOs may partially or completely move. Other potential new lines of activity are community- or employer-based wellness programs, occupational health services (e.g., Rhode Island Group Health Association), and private utilization review (e.g., Physicians Health Plan in Minnesota). HMOs with significant elderly enrollments may also begin providing and/or arranging for an expanded number of long-term and social support services. The Health Care Financing Administration is already funding demonstration projects at several social HMO sites, which will provide a broad range of health and social services on a cost-efficient prospectively budgeted basis for elderly populations (e.g., Group Health Plan in Minneapolis and the Kaiser plan in Portland).

As individual HMO plans become larger, they will be better able to negotiate more favorable hospital agreements. These agreements will take a variety of forms, including discounted per diem or charge structures, comprehensive per admission or per member (capitation) payments, and various risk sharing provisions. Very large plans (100,000 or more enrollees) will increasingly acquire their own hospitals. The incentives to acquire such facilities will be further heightened if state rate-setting programs adopt provisions limiting the ability of HMOs to negotiate discounts with community facilities.

Operational and selection procedures for PPOs will have to move toward practice patterns and utilization profiles as the primary criteria if PPOs are to be successful. Relying on discounts as a long-range (or even short-range) measurement of cost-effectiveness is illusionary. Slight variations in treatment intensities on the part of the physician can easily make up for the discount.

Last but not least, we foresee a melding of different forms of insurance and alternative delivery systems, which will make neat definitions even more elusive, other than as descriptions of prototypes. More HMOs will probably use experience rating rather than community rating, both to compete with other plans and to meet demand from employers who find that their healthy employees enroll in HMOs disproportionately. Greater cost-sharing in HMOs is also likely adding consumer incentives for efficiency. Some HMOs may waive the lock-in, allowing patients to use any provider, but with cost-sharing disincentives for using nonparticipating providers.

We also expect to see PPOs that share financially in the risk. One legal issue is the point at which they require licensure as either an insurer or an HMO. Insurers themselves may come to adopt incentives to use particular providers, including using selected primary care physicians as case managers.

DESIGNING VIABLE ALTERNATIVE DELIVERY SYSTEMS

An HMO, whether for profit or not, must generate sufficient income in the long run to meet its operating costs and provide a reasonable return on investment. PPOs entail a much lower financial investment and thus can fail without creating the same level of burden for sponsors or patients. Although there is no "cookbook" for HMO, let alone for PPO, success or failure, analyses of past HMO financial problems can serve to identify several important factors. These include adequate capitalization, capable leadership, market acceptance, and provider support.

While some of the important features that characterize successful HMOs can be documented, for PPOs they are somewhat speculative. PPOs differ from PIPPs in two principle respects: the absence of the lock-in and the risk being borne by the purchaser, not the PPO. Both organizations typically encompass a multiplicity of providers who, as individual persons or entities, have incentives to increase volume. Beyond that, the similarities outweigh the differences. Thus, it is instructive to understand both the parallels, where they exist, and the differences.

Capitalization

Every new business requires the infusion of capital to finance start-up costs (planning, development, marketing, staffing, etc.), and most, including HMOs, face an initial period of operating at a loss. Once breakeven is achieved, the plan can begin to generate surpluses to pay off debts and finance future expansions, renovations, acquisitions, and so forth. Internally generated surpluses are often insufficient to react fully to these opportunities and needs, and even mature plans often must turn to external sources of capital. In contrast, the capital requirements of a PPO are usually minimal.

Capable Leadership

An HMO incorporates a complex set of interrelated financial, medical, and marketing objectives. Implementing marketing and/or delivery system strategies without due consideration for their impact on plan finances (or on each other) has often been disastrous. It is essential, therefore, that the plan be directed by a manager who has both a strong business acumen and strong "people" skills and, thus, can bring about the necessary internal coordination. The policy-making board should share these convictions and capabilities, as well as be influential in economic and political circles. Board members must especially appreciate that hopes of equity, quality, or affordability cannot be realized in the absence of a sound financial operation. Although typically the PPO has a simpler structure, it too requires capable leadership to address such issues as provider and purchaser relations, data systems, and utilization review.

Marketing

An HMO needs an adequate enrollment base to break even. Since most HMO enrollment is obtained through employee and union groups, the plan must be accepted both by the individuals eligible through these groups and by the officials who determine which health plan options to offer and how to represent them to the work force.

An environment providing a variety of medium to large sized groups is favorable because it facilitates economical marketing and, at the same time, minimizes the risk of "make or break" situations with any single employer. It is also helpful to have benefit decisions made locally, so that there is access to decision makers. Indemnity health insurance plans that are comprehensive are favorable also, because the HMO is likely to attract less healthy enrollees if the employee's contribution to the HMO is much greater than his contribution to the indemnity plan.

Employers' knowledge and support of HMOs are important factors, since most people learn about health plans through their employers. Employers can lend support by allowing access to the work force for marketing presentations and by offering more than one HMO, as well as by willingness to contribute equally to insurance and HMO premiums.

Most markets will be well-positioned on some of these factors and not others. Recent research has confirmed that some of these variables may support the establishment of the first HMO in a community but restrain aggregate HMO market growth (Morrisey and Ashby 1982). Moreover, many of these factors are matters of degree rather than being totally absent or present. Thus, most SMSAs can support some level of HMO activity.

Marketing will also be a key to PPO success, mostly in terms of demonstrating to carriers and purchasers that the PPO has a viable product. Both business and union leaders are concerned that they not channel enrollees to providers whose quality of care is questionable. Beyond that, the PPO will have to demonstrate that it is, or has the potential to be, efficient. In this regard, it is important to note that the PPO can affect purchasers' costs in four ways. First, the discount saves money relative to the usual charges of the participating provider. Second, any reduction in cost-sharing results in higher benefit payments. Third, the reduction of out-of-pocket expenses to the consumer in the absence of utilization controls can be expected to generate increased utilization, which also increases benefit payments. Finally, the preferred providers themselves may be either expensive or reasonably priced, and the shifting of patients among providers will impact on plan cost. It is the net effect of these four factors that determines the ultimate cost impact on the purchaser.

Provider Relations

In order to attract and retain enrollees, an HMO must provide an acceptable style (quality and volume) of health care at a competitive premium. In addition, given the comprehensive services that the plan is obligated to underwrite, the HMO must be able to control utilization rates and prices.

As the largest category of expenditures, inpatient hospital care is the key target of cost control. HMOs usually incorporate a variety of strategies, including: the selection of physicians who are not overly prone to hospitalize, informal peer interaction and formal utilization review, benefit structures that remove financial barriers to out-of-hospital treatment, administrative strategies (e.g., preadmission and length-of-stay certifications), risk-and-incentive reimbursement systems, the provision of lifestyle education and preventive intervention services to enrollees, utilization of lower cost facilities, and negotiation of favorable price agreements.

It is in the area of provider relations that the lessons for PPOs from PIPPs are perhaps the most relevant. Many PIPPs in their early years neither select participating providers carefully nor monitor physician practice patterns. The result, commonly, is that the intended efficiencies of prepayment are not achieved, resulting in financial problems for the PIPP. At that point, the organization is forced to select providers more carefully and institute tough utilization controls if it is to continue to operate. Examples of HMOs that have experienced this cycle are CompreCare in Denver and Physicians Health Plan in Minnesota. Similarly, the successful PPO will have to select providers carefully and demonstrate that it has internal controls on physician practice patterns that overcome the incentives on individual practitioners to increase volume. A purchaser considering a contract with a PPO would be well advised to make sure that adequate selection process and delivery system controls are in place, and that data will be available for program evaluation over time.

REFERENCES

Bryant, B. E., and J. Boscarino. "Rising Costs Concern Physicians." *American Medical News* (23 November 1979):1–2.

Carroll, M. S., and R. H. Arnett III. "Private Health Insurance Plans in 1978 and 1979: A Review of Coverage, Enrollment, and Financial Experience." *Health Care Financing Review* 3(September 1981):55–87.

Fox, P. D., and E. J. Tell. *Private Sector Health Care Initiatives: A Case Study of the Denver Area.* Washington, D.C.: Lewin and Associates, Inc., 1983.

InterStudy. 1983. *National HMO Census, 1982.* Excelsior, Minn.

Louis Harris and Associates. *Employers and HMO's: A Nationwide Survey of Corporate Employers in Areas Served by Health Maintenance Organizations.* Menlo Park, Calif.: Henry J. Kaiser Family Foundation, 1980.

————. *Medical Practice in the 1980s: Physicians Look at Their Changing Profession.* Menlo Park, Calif.: Henry J. Kaiser Family Foundation, 1982.

Luft, H. S. *Health Maintenance Organizations: Dimensions of Performance.* New York: John Wiley & Sons, 1981.

Morrisey, M., and C. Ashby. "An Empirical Analysis of HMO Market Share." *Inquiry* 19(Summer 1982):136–149.

Shadle, M. *National HMO Firms, 1983.* Excelsior, Minn.: InterStudy, 1983.

"Sharp Rise Seen in U.S. Medical Groups." *American Medical News* (29 January 1982):7–8.

4

Utilization Review

Andrew Webber and
Willis B. Goldbeck

INTRODUCTION

The medical care cost increases of recent years have fueled demands for accountability from purchasers and have focused attention on utilization review (UR). In addition, the advent of hospital prospective reimbursement has placed new emphasis on the need to change physician practice patterns. Thus, UR is becoming increasingly accepted as the method by which quality and cost effectiveness are advanced and vigilantly monitored.

Rewarding cost-effective medical intervention, always implicit in prepaid systems, is now spreading to the fee-for-service sector. Physicians in traditional practice are feeling the pinch of reimbursement reform, alternative delivery systems, and an oversupply of doctors. Competition for patients is intensifying. Albeit largely a defensive strategy, UR within the fee-for-service sector becomes a method of protecting market share and responding to purchaser demands for accountability. There is a growing understanding that UR is in the long-term interests of the fee-for-service physician community.

However, the driving force behind the UR movement has become the private employer frustrated by seemingly endless premium increases and encouraged by the growing awareness that UR is a precursor to a wide range of cost-management efforts. The ability to profile provider-specific utilization experience is the starting point for other stages of UR and can serve to identify apparently inappropriate utilization. This ability gives the purchaser parity in discussions with the provider community and is essential for any negotiated (or preferred) provider agreements. Concurrent UR and preadmission review can be targeted for maximum return on investment. Benefits can be redesigned. Worksite wellness programs can be established in response to particular illness patterns. Finally, efficient providers can be selected and rewarded with increased patient volume.

This chapter describes the evolving nature of UR and some emerging issues pertaining to it. The next section defines UR and describes the elements in the review process. The third reports on private sector UR initiatives of purchasers, fiscal intermediaries, peer review, consulting, and academic organizations. The fourth section discusses emerging issues pertaining to data access and disclosure, the cost impact of UR, consideration of who is to perform UR, and the likely evolution of the next generation of UR mechanisms.

UTILIZATION REVIEW—WHAT IT DOES

Background

UR is the process of assessing medical care services to assure quality, medical necessity, and appropriateness in terms of level of care and locus of treatment. Historically, UR efforts have been focused on quality assurance through the self-policing of the medical profession (e.g., hospital teaching committees). Quality assurance has involved the participation of various public and private entities and has been accomplished through professional licensure, control of hospital privileges, specialty certification, and voluntary peer review activities. The traditional orientation towards quality assurance as the primary thrust of UR activities was reflected in the efforts of state licensing boards, the establishment of foundations for medical care, hospital UR committees, the medical industry's creation of the Joint Committee on the Accreditation of Hospitals (JCAH), and the federal government's original (1966) UR requirements for Medicare and Medicaid.

As part of the 1972 Social Security Act amendments, the professional standards review organization (PSRO) program was established. The PSRO mandate was to assure that Medicare paid only for care that was medically necessary and that conformed to professional standards of quality. The nation was divided into 195 PSRO regions, and by 1980 nearly two-thirds of the nation's hospitals were under

PSRO review. However, the PSROs were in trouble even before many were officially designated. The AMA and many local medical societies opposed them; government financial support never matched the operational requirements; private sector review was virtually unheard of; there was considerable skepticism of the value of allowing the profession to police itself; and the program lacked clear objectives that lent themselves to evaluation.

With this background it is not surprising that PSRO evaluations were neither definitive nor consistent. By the late 1970s it became clear that the move toward deregulation, coupled with the lack of substantial evidence proving PSRO cost-effectiveness, signaled the demise of the original PSRO program. From 1979–1983 the program received diminished support and was legislatively replaced by the peer review organizations (PROs), effective 1984. The PROs would be performance-judged organizations that competed for government contracts, rather than receiving grants, and would likely have to conduct private review to survive.

In the past decade more and more evidence has confirmed purchasers' suspicions that much care is of questionable necessity. The indices of questionable utilization that have received the greatest attention relate to variations in hospitalization rates. Although most striking when comparing fee-for-service to prepaid plans (Weisinger et al. 1976, Perrott 1971), the variance in utilization is also apparent within the traditional fee-for-service sector. Studies comparing east to west coast hospital use rates show large discrepancies that cannot be medically explained (Blumberg 1981).

In Iowa, Wennberg's research found problems comparable to those identified in New England. Hospital admissions across comparable areas varied from 109 to 238 per 1,000; prostate surgery admissions varied nearly fourfold; and admissions for tonsillectomies varied fivefold. This analysis contributed directly to the decision of employers, labor, and the planning agency to make the reduction of excess hospital utilization Iowa's top cost-management priority. Private employer contracts with the PSROs increased, and so began in Iowa an evolving cost-management strategy with UR at its core. More generally, Professor Wennberg's studies have concluded that there is often "no relationship between clinical need and intensity of service." Variations are explained by physician supply, hospital bed supply, inpatient third-party payment incentives, and the practice styles physicians learned during medical school and residencies (Wennberg and Gittelsohn 1982).

Also, inappropriate use of hospital ancillary services has been documented. Studies show that lab and x-ray services are routinely ordered despite the knowledge that they will not contribute to a patient's diagnosis. Often, results are not even read by the attending physician (Dixon and Lazlo 1974, Griner and Liptzin 1971).

Today, the dual objective for UR is to eliminate inappropriate and clinically unjustified medical care services while preserving quality. There is a perceived tension between these two objectives that has made UR controversial. Providers have often criticized purchasers for their single-minded attention to cost cutting, and purchasers have blamed providers for hiding behind concern for quality to justify a failure to focus attention on inappropriate or unnecessary services.

How Utilization Review Works

There are many different forms of UR. This chapter explores those related most prominently to private sector initiatives: profile analysis, concurrent review, preadmission review, and quality review. The focus to date has largely been on inpatient hospital acute care. With the exception of dental, worker's compensation, and some mental health services, ambulatory care review is rarely performed.

Two areas are not discussed: claims auditing and coverage policy. Claims auditing entails determining whether payment is justified, using as criteria factors other than medical necessity. Claims are reviewed to verify that the claimant is eligible for payment, that the benefit for which payment is claimed is covered, that the benefit is not payable under another policy, and that the service billed was in fact rendered.

Coverage policy can be described as the identification of procedures or services that should virtually never be reimbursed because they are rarely, if ever, efficacious or because alternative interventions exist. For example, certain procedures may be judged obsolete because of medical advances. Others may be judged potentially acceptable only under specific cirumstances. The Medical Necessity Project of the Blue Cross/Blue Shield Association is the most prominent private sector example of an effort to terminate coverage of procedures or services that are not efficacious.

Profile analysis

Profile analysis is the logical first step in a UR strategy and is the method by which problem areas are identified and subsequent review activity focused or targeted. Profiles are statistical reports on provider-specific utilization patterns for patients who have been classified into clinically meaningful groups based on such factors as diagnosis, age, and sex. Each group is assumed to be homogeneous in terms of expected resource consumption. Comparisons and evaluations of the utilization patterns can then be made. The use of diagnosis-related groups (DRGs), developed originally as a research tool at Yale University by Professor John Thompson, is the most prominent system now being used to generate profiles of resources consumed once a patient is admitted to the hospital. In addition to being the basis for reimbursement in the new Medicare prospective pricing system, the DRG method of analysis is being sold commercially to private purchasers, insurance carriers, and third-party administrators.

An alternative profiling method, the Appropriateness Evaluation Protocol (AEP), has been developed by the Health Data Institute in Boston. AEP entails assigning nurses to hospitals to determine the necessity of admission and expected days of care based on 27 objective criteria applicable to all adult medical, surgical, and gynecological patients in acute care hospitals. Days not meeting the criteria are identified for feedback to purchasers, fiscal intermediaries, hospital review committees, peer review organizations, and practicing physicians. Physician-specific profiles of potentially unnecessary days can be generated. The Delmarva Foundation for Medical Care, a Maryland PSRO, has modified the AEP instrument with impressive results. Rather than relying on physician judgment to determine the appropriateness of a hospital day, this PSRO developed a nonacute profile (NAP) that requires the application of specific utilization criteria. Furthermore, the data method developed permits application of the system to physicians rather than just hospitals. The profile has been particularly effective in reducing nonacute days at the end of hospital stays, depending on the time of year (patients were more willing to go home early in summer than winter). Both the DRG and the AEP approaches were developed with research funding from the federal government. In fact, the evolution of private UR has evolved in no small measure from the federal investment in the PSRO program.

The awakening purchaser recognition of the need for accurate utilization and cost data upon which to base cost-management strategies is often frustrated not only by provider reluctance to provide the information but also by the poor quality of the data. Medical records are notorious for inaccuracies, illegible physician penmanship, and significant delays between discharge and completion. Other problems are evidenced by carriers reporting that between 30 percent and 80 percent of all hospital bills contain at least one inaccuracy (the National Academy of Sciences found a 40 percent error rate), although some errors are more serious than others. The discharge abstracts are another source of error. Clinically meaningful information is often reported in narrative rather than coded form. Some carriers use their own codes rather than the ICD-9-CM, which the federal government and many purchasers support as the standard diagnostic code, thus further complicating the process of comparing providers. Employers are aware of the data quality problems but realize that improved medical record keeping, more meaningful claims information, and reduced error rates will result from the serious application of the data by purchasers to reimbursement policy.

Medicare's new prospective pricing system, with its reliance on DRGs, is seen by many employers as alleviating the comparability problem. The need to present data by DRGs gives hospitals strong incentives to upgrade the quality of their data, incentives which are enhanced as private payers also begin to use such data. Also, per case reimbursement under Medicare results in incentives for reduced utilization of ancillaries and increased admissions, but it also increases the importance of PSROs and other UR groups conducting effective admission review in addition to their traditional length-of-stay review function.

Concurrent review

Concurrent review addresses the medical necessity and appropriateness of hospital admissions and continued stays. It is conducted while a patient is in the hospital and is usually performed by a nurse under the supervision of a physician advisor. The private sector purchaser typically pays between $10 and $30 per review. These reviews often become the basis for physician profiles.

Shortly after admission, the hospital admitting office provides the review organization with notification of admission and an admitting diagnosis. Often an actual review of the medical record is performed. Based on diagnosis-specific criteria, an initial length of stay is assigned and becomes a checkpoint for further review. The criteria are usually based on statistics on the distribution of length of stay by diagnosis and age for the United States and each region. The most widely used statistics are those generated by the Commission on Professional and Hospital Activities (see next section).

Concurrent review has been the principal activity of the PSRO program. These physician-based organizations, traditionally reluctant to go beyond their legislative mandate to review public program patients, have more recently demonstrated a growing interest in contracting with purchasers for concurrent review of private patients, in part to expand their revenue base in light of what they perceive of as inadequate federal funding. Insurance carriers, individual companies, and increasingly, multiemployer groups have signed concurrent review contracts with PSROs.

The cost-benefit ratio of investment in concurrent review has been widely debated. Evaluations have not been performed with control groups and with a duration sufficient to capture the impact on systemwide costs, utilization by other payers, or changes in the structure of the delivery system (bed reduction, replacement or additive services, etc.). Nonetheless, results of concurrent review programs, as reported by respected employers such as Deere and Caterpillar, have led other employers to support the concept while accepting the uncertainties regarding the long range impact. For example, Deere reports that, in four and one-half years, hospital days per 1,000 were reduced by 31.2 percent in Iowa and 35.6 percent in Ilinois, resulting in a ten- to fifteenfold return on their investment in PSRO contracts.

Preadmission review

Preadmission review is the process of verifying the medical necessity and appropriateness of a hospital stay prior to admission. It is the second most emotionally charged issue, after disclosure of provider-specific utilization data, that has come between purchasers and providers in the UR field. One argument in favor of preadmission over concurrent review is that an inappropriate hospitalization is best prevented prior to admission. Both hospitals and physicians have strongly resisted the notion of preadmission review, complaining of inappropriate and burdensome oversight and fearing loss of patient volume. The extent to which preadmission review is growing in popularity can be seen in the work of the San Francisco Peer Review Organization, Inc., which currently has contracts with Levi Strauss, Bechtel, Crown Zellerbach, Bank of America, the San Francisco Department of Public Health, and the Record Factory. The scope of review ranges from all elective surgery to only a select list of elective procedures. Similar programs are conducted by other PSROs (e.g., Colorado Foundation for Medical Care, Delaware Review Organization, and the Mid-State Foundation for Medical Care in Peoria) and by non-PSRO UR companies, such as Co-Med in Columbus, Ohio.

Quality review

Traditionally, medical care evaluation studies or medical audits, as they are sometimes called, have been the leading activity under the rubric of quality review. They consist of in-depth reviews of medical records as a way of analyzing the quality and nature of selected health care services rendered in hospitals. The PSRO program and the JCAH require that medical care evaluation studies be conducted and that one such study be in progress at all times, although their effect on patient care or health status has not been systematically studied.

For the purchaser of care, the goal of quality review is to determine the efficacy of medical intervention. Efficacy, unlike efficiency, is concerned with patient health outcomes rather than whether services were rendered in an appropriate and fiscally disciplined manner. This is not to imply that efficiency and efficacy are incompatible; it might very well be discovered that the highest quality patient health outcome is produced by a service that is delivered in a cost-effective manner. Excess use and unnecessary services not only are inefficient but also add to the risk inherent in all medical care.

The challenge to the medical research community is to rank severity of illness at the start of medical intervention and be able to predict health outcome with some range of accuracy. Actual health outcomes can then be measured against expected or desired health outcomes, and the efficacy of medical intervention can be determined. Ultimately, purchasers can identify and reward efficacy, and a balance with efficiency can be struck.

This kind of quality review profiling is in its infancy but is being researched. Building severity of illness into DRGs is the first step. Research by Susan Horn at Johns Hopkins University and Charles Jacobs at Interqual is directed at developing a system to assure that patients in a DRG category are truly homogeneous in terms of predicted resource consumption and final health outcome.

Other examples include the work of Dr. Richard Egdahl at Boston University to identify the most efficient and effective physician practice patterns and the evolution of U.S. Administrators' model treatment plans into outcome standards validated by panels of nationally recognized physicians. These are discussed further in the next section.

UTILIZATION REVIEW—WHO DOES IT?

As recently as five years ago, listing all significant private review activities outside of the hospital's own programs would have been easy. Today, the level of activity is so great that reporting the full range of private sector initiatives is impossible. By providing examples of private sector initiatives, this section offers a sense of what is happening and who some of the key players are. It discusses activities of purchasers, fiscal intermediaries, peer review organizations, consultants/entrepreneurs, and academics.

Purchasers

The interest of purchasers in UR has risen in tandem with their interest in constraining the rise in medical care costs. Their demands for better information from hospitals and for cost and utilization reports from fiscal intermediaries are becoming more frequent and increasing in sophistication. Deere & Company and American Telephone and Telegraph (AT&T) are examples of companies at the forefront of UR activities, including relying on UR information to develop a more comprehensive cost-management strategy.

In 1971, Deere & Company made the decision to develop a self-funded and self-administered benefits program. In 1977, Deere installed a claims processing system, entitled Comprehensive Insurance Claims Handling (CINCH), which specifies the data that providers must report on a claims form before payment will be made. Deere captures the following information:

— diagnosis code by ICD-9-CM
— procedure code by CPT-4
— provider of service code
— patient data (name and address, social security number, age, sex)
— claim type code (hospital, medical, dental, etc.)
— dates of treatment
— amount charged
— amount denied and reason code
— amount paid and date paid
— Medicare eligibility
— coordination of benefit information

From this information, Deere has derived cost and utilization profiles on a provider-specific basis, and PSROs under contract to conduct concurrent review have been directed to focus on problem areas. Deere health insurance benefits are being redesigned as claims profiles uncover procedures that, commonly, can safely and less expensively be performed on an outpatient basis. A wellness program is being developed in response to identified needs. Cost and utilization profiles also represented the factual base for discussions with the provider community on the establishment of two HMOs.

AT&T developed its own data specifications that are required of all carriers with which it contracts, although full implementation has not yet been completed. The specifications capture all the data elements that Deere collects. Each transaction generates a record containing information regarding patient demographics, services rendered, and diagnosis. A key aspect of the system is the ability to link multiple records, even from two or more carriers, to create a single claim record. Results to date are encouraging, and the company expects the data to become the centerpiece of its cost-management, health planning, and benefit redesign efforts in the years ahead.

The Business Roundtable (BRT) has made data requirements a primary focus of its Health Initiatives Project. In 1982 meetings were convened of senior representatives of national hospital, physician, insurance, business and labor groups to discuss data issues. AT&T outlined its data specifications, and in May 1983 the BRT Health Initiatives Project held regional seminars to educate employer representatives about the AT&T model and why they might want to adopt it for their own use. BRT surveys indicate that the need for a common data system was one of industry's highest priorities, and the Health Initiatives Project now encourages BRT members to adopt—or adapt—the AT&T model.

The Washington Business Group on Health (WBGH) supports uniformity in claims data and full disclosure of pricing information. For example, in testimony on Medicare DRG reimbursement, WBGH called for implementation of the Uniform Bill 82 (UB–82). UB–82, developed by the Health Care Financing Administration, would ensure that certain data elements were entered on all hospital claim forms, regardless of payer. On the local level, WBGH has worked with member companies and coalitions on the design of data systems, claims and cost-management strategies, and state legislation that would promote the accountability objectives of the purchasers.

In April 1983, the implementation of UB–82 was legislatively mandated for all Iowa hospitals. Purchaser leadership in Iowa—including Deere, Pioneer Hi-Bred, Meredith Corporation, and the *Des Moines Tribune and Register*—aggressively lobbied for the new law, which creates a statewide data clearinghouse that will allow individual purchasers to access utilization and price profiles of their employees.

Purchaser coalitions around the country have also placed a high priority on better claims information to facilitate profile analysis.

— First among the coalitions to make data a priority was PENJERDEL in Philadelphia. Hospital comparative data reports have been generated for the past several years, and in 1982 this effort was expanded to include physician utilization.

— The Midwest Business Group on Health has created nine user groups, which are comprised of coalition members that contract with the same insurance carrier. Members of a user group work with the fiscal intermediary to develop uniform data elements and upgrade claims management and analysis. Profiles are generated for individual members and can then be compared to others in the user group.

— The South Florida Health Action Coalition in Miami has also made profile analysis a priority. Price and utilization profiles that are provider-specific are constructed for individual members and then aggregated for the entire coalition.

— The Fairfield-Westchester Coalition in New York has established a separate data consortium.

Coalitions have also stimulated multiemployer review efforts. Although most of these initiatives are still in the planning stages, some already report positive results:

— A communitywide private review program of both preadmission and concurrent review was initiated in Phoenix, Arizona in the early 1970s, involving 75 employers. Entitled the Certified Hospital Admission Program (CHAP) and conducted by the Maricopa County Medical Foundation, the effort has yielded significant results. Motorola, Inc., the driving purchaser behind the efforts, reports having reduced its average length of stay from 7.5 to 5.6 days, and its hospital days from 535 to 422 per 1,000 enrollees.

— The Minnesota Coalition on Health Care Costs in Minneapolis helped foster a communitywide private review effort starting in July 1981. Sixteen major purchasers—including General Mills, Honeywell, Control Data, 3M, and Pillsbury—contracted with the Minnesota Foundation for Health Care Evaluation to conduct concurrent review as well as preadmission review for selected procedures. The foundation is currently reviewing the hospital care of roughly 140,000 insureds in a seven-county metropolitan area.

In the last year, the communities of San Diego, Cleveland, Kansas City, and, most recently, Toledo and Chicago, have developed UR programs involving multiple purchasers. All were stimulated by local coalitions.

Profile analysis performed by peer review organizations has been another important avenue for purchasers. Peer review organizations have increasingly become a critical source of information on purchaser utilization experience, in part because of their access to hospital discharge abstracts. Examples of corporate relationships with peer review organizations include the following:

— Du Pont, at its headquarters in Wilmington, has signed a private review contract with a PSRO, the Delaware Review Organization, in which concurrent review will be conducted, but only after profile analysis has been completed to identify problem areas.

— Caterpillar Tractor Company in Peoria, Illinois, contracted with the Mid-State Foundation for Medical Care. It has reported, over a four-year period, decreases of 10 percent in admission rates and 8 percent in average length of stay, yielding a reduction of 17 percent in days of care per 1,000 enrollees.

— In Milwaukee, Wisconsin, the Foundation for Medical Care Evaluation of Southeastern Wisconsin has signed individual review contracts with such employers as A. O. Smith, Allis-Chalmers, and Briggs and Stratton, all of which report cost savings. A. O. Smith, for example, reports reducing its hospital utilization rate from 874 to 535 days per 1,000, just a year and a half after review was initiated.

— Sundstrand Corporation, in Rockford, Illinois, first signed a private review contract with the local peer review organization in 1978 and, over a four-year period, witnessed its days per 1,000 decrease from 747 to 552.

Carriers and Fiscal Intermediaries

Some contend that carriers have traditionally played a passive role in private sector UR initiatives, reflecting in large measure the expectations of purchasers, who were unwilling to pay for UR. Only recently have purchaser demands induced carriers to exert greater effort, and in the future it is likely that those that cannot demonstrate their ability to profile utilization patterns and develop strategies to control inappropriate use of services will lose business. It should be noted that, even when employers self-insure, the role of the fiscal intermediary as claims processor continues to be important, except for firms that also self-administer. Thus, for all but a small percentage of employers, carriers and fiscal intermediaries are the primary source of utilization and price information.

Commercial carriers

Health insurance carriers are responding to purchase requests for more information. One result has been the establishment of new relationships with data firms that have profiling capabilities.

At the beginning of 1980, John Hancock Mutual Life Insurance Company acquired the product lines and resources that constituted the health care information system and services business of Dikewood Industries, Inc. A subsidiary company was formed entitled Hancock/Dikewood Services, Inc. In Milwaukee, Hancock has signed a contract with the Foundation for Medical Care Evaluation of Southeastern Wisconsin to provide concurrent review for 2,400 of its enrollees.

In early 1983, Metropolitan Life Insurance Company bought a DRG data analysis firm, Corporate Health Strategies, and in the same year CIGNA Corporation bought a minority interest in Health Systems International, another DRG data firm, which evolved from the research team at Yale that first developed DRGs.

In addition, the Health Insurance Association of America (HIAA) has created a task force on data issues to respond to policyholder and coalition requests for better information. In December 1982, the HIAA task force recommended that its member companies adopt a standard data set for hospital inpatient data. One criticism of the HIAA approach is that diagnoses are to be reported by only 18 categories, which many view as too few in number and not compatible with DRGs.

HIAA has publicly supported the PSRO program, and one of its leading members, CIGNA, was instrumental in lobbying for enactment of the Peer Review Improvement Act, which was enacted in 1982 as part of the Tax Equity and Fiscal Responsibility Act and authorized the peer review organization (PROs), which are successor organizations to the PSROs. CIGNA's support, much like that of other members of the Washington Business Group on Health, was based on the positive results generated by private review. CIGNA performed an internal study of the impact on premium costs of health planning, all-party payment systems, and contracts with peer review organizations. Peer review contracts were found to yield the greatest return on CIGNA's investment. CIGNA has signed contracts with the Washington State PSRO and the Hartford County PSRO.

The commercial carriers have little internal capacity to do concurrent or preadmission review, but they have selectively signed contracts with peer review organizations. In this regard, they are much like purchasers, who have sought relationships with these organizations.

Blue Cross/Blue Shield

The demand for better data on utilization experience, particularly from national accounts such as IBM, General Motors, and General Electric, has stimulated the Blues to respond. A major problem for the Blues (as well as other) plans in developing utilization profiles has been the absence of procedure information on hospital (Blue Cross) claims. Typically, procedure information is found only on physician (Blue Shield) claim forms. Furthermore, the task of merging hospital and physician data is a difficult one.

Many Blue Cross plans have worked closely with the Health Data Institute to develop better profiling of provider utilization patterns. Some 30 plans have conducted training sessions in 1983 to implement the Appropriateness Evaluation Protocol discussed in the previous section. This represents a serious and concerted effort to develop a strong profiling base that will help protect market share and respond to purchaser demands.

Traditionally, the Blues have not generally been supportive of separate peer review organizations. Although roughly 15 Blues plans around the country have contracted with peer review organizations, the posture of the national association has been neutral, reflecting skepticism of the PSRO program. The Blues, as the predominant fiscal intermediary for Medicare, have argued that they can perform UR of Medicare beneficiaries more effectively than the peer review organizations. They will have the opportunity to prove this contention under the new PRO program, which, in those areas where peer review groups have not met performance standards, authorizes the federal government to contract with a fiscal intermediary.

Third-party administrators

As self-insurance has increased, so have the number of third-party administrators, i.e., firms that process claims for self-insuring groups but that are not licensed as insurers. Many have developed a market niche by emphasizing rapid payment and careful claims auditing, and a few have created UR programs. One of the more innovative and aggressive is U.S. Administrators, headquartered in California.

At U.S. Administrators, nationally prominent physicians serve as consultants and help to develop and continually update a series of computerized model treatment screens for specific diagnostic codes. Any discrepancy between services rendered and what is deemed appropriate by the treatment screen is flagged for analysis while the claim is being processed, often leading to denial of payment. If the provider challenges a payment decision, U.S. Administrators will defend its analysis, in court if necessary.

When a patient enters the hospital, hospital staff are expected to complete and file a predetermination form that requests the admitting diagnosis and identification of the attending physicians. (Failure to do so can result in reimbursement being denied.) Upon receipt of a diagnosis, an appropriate length of stay is assigned based on the model treatment screens and transmitted on the same day to the hospital, attending physician, and individual patient. Subsequently, if a hospital bill is received that deviates from the length of stay determination, the excess days will not be reimbursed until additional clinical justification is received from the provider. If the excess days still cannot be justified, payment is denied, and the patient is held harmless. Using this method, U.S. Administrators reports being able to reduce length of stay for its clients by approximately 20 percent. It also reports savings from ancillary service review and dental plan predetermination controls.

Peer Review Organizations

Peer review organizations (Foundations for Medical Care—organizations typically established by medical societies to do private review—and PSROs) have had the dubious distinction of continually having to explain their existence in response to questions regarding their motivation for serious UR activity. There are enough isolated examples, however, of effective peer review organizations to justify the efforts of some of these groups, particularly those with strong physician leadership, technical capabilities, and access to meaningful hospital information.

The more enterprising peer review organizations have entered the private market with enthusiasm. For example, the Iowa Foundation for Medical Care (IFMC) has developed the largest private review business in the country. Partly stimulated by the interests of Deere & Company, 80 percent of the private health insurance market in Iowa has contracted for concurrent or preadmission review for selected procedures. IFMC has also created a business advisory committee, a vehicle through which purchaser concerns can be communicated. Another example is the Foundation for Medical Care Evaluation of Southeastern Wisconsin, which, through contracts with purchasers and fiscal intermediaries, conducts private review for over 700 employers.

A survey conducted in 1982 by the American Medical Peer Review Association (AMPRA), the national association of PSROs, found that 75 of the 142 PSROs surveyed reported having signed contracts for private review, and an additional 16 stated they were in the process of negotiating such contracts. A number of forces—the uncertainty of federal funding, the growing interests of the purchaser community, and the acknowledgement that greater competition for patients will place a premium on demonstrating efficiency in health service delivery—all converge to motivate peer review organizations to seek private review contracts.

Consulting Firms and Universities

A substantial number of private firms have entered the field in response to the growing demand for UR. Some have origins in the academic community; others spring from the computer and data-processing world; and still others have been, or are presently, affiliated with peer review organizations. These firms work with purchasers, fiscal intermediaries, and PSROs to profile utilization patterns and identify opportunities for cost-management. Many specialize in developing DRG profiles. Among the DRG profile firms and UR consultants are Corporate Health Strategies, the Commons Management Group, Puter Associates, the 2M Group, Medstat, Interqual, and the Health Data Institute. These firms have generally worked at single locations rather than providing services for multilocation employers.

There are also many data-processing firms that conduct UR. They predominantly serve peer review organizations and hospitals. The oldest and best known is the Commission on Professional and Hospital Activities (CPHA), a nonprofit organization supported by the American Hospital Association. It developed the Professional Activity Summary (PAS), a shared computer medical record information system that compares average lengths of stay, number and types of tests used, and autopsy rates for given diagnostic conditions. PAS is often used to assign length-of-stay benchmarks for concurrent review. Commonwealth of Charlottesville, another data processor, has contracts with 30 PSROs.

Responding to the need of multilocation employers to avoid having to negotiate many separate review contracts, several firms are offering a review network approach. Health Care COMPR Corp. in Joliet, Illinois, markets a range of UR products to individual purchasers and fiscal intermediaries. A. S. Hansen, Inc. has joined with SysteMetrics, a subsidiary of Data Resources, Inc. (DRI), to combine DRG analysis with cost analysis and an approach called disease staging. Co-Med, in Columbus, Ohio, is a physician-funded organization that has established a reputation for changing physician practice patterns based on utilization analysis. Medical Review Inc. (MRI) in Milburn, New Jersey, has signed contracts with the stock brokerage firm of Paine, Webber, Jackson, Curtis, Inc. and the retail chain Associated Dry Goods, to perform concurrent review work in multisite locations.

University research and academic centers have been the source of many innovations in UR. Yale University is the home of diagnosis related groups. DRGs were developed in the early 1970s, originally as a research tool for quality assurance and UR activities in hospital settings. DRGs are a patient classification scheme that groups patients into homogeneous categories with respect to specific dignostic, therapeutic, and demographic characteristics. The objective is to define hospital products by grouping similar patients so that true utilization and cost comparisons can be performed. While originally developed as a utilization tool, DRGs have been adopted by New Jersey and, most recently, the Medicare program as the unit of payment for hospital reimbursement.

Boston University's Center for Industry and Health Care has become an innovator in utilization management. The Center has been active in data and profile analysis and has contracts with ALCOA, DuPont, and Armco to work with physicians. In a nonadversarial fashion, but with the assistance of the corporation as leverage, center staff gain access to hospital discharge abstracts and conduct a utilization profile. Problem areas are identified. A process of communication with area physicians is then initiated.

Staff at the Center for Hospital Finance and Management at Johns Hopkins University have performed extensive research in case-mix measurements. They have sought to demonstrate that DRGs are an innovative but presently unrefined system in one principal aspect: they fail to build in a factor to reflect severity of illness. As a result, they contend that use of DRGs is inequitable for reimbursement purposes; those hospitals with a sicker patient case-mix will be inadequately reimbursed, whereas a less severely ill patient case-mix represents a financial windfall to other institutions.

EMERGING ISSUES IN UTILIZATION REVIEW

As the dialogue in the private sector begins in earnest, issues are emerging that will challenge purchasers and providers.

Information Access and Disclosure

For those who believe in a more competitive medical marketplace, as many purchasers do, the combination of information access and disclosure becomes a key. However, access to, and disclosure of, medical record information, which is the best basis for accurate utilization profiling, is an emotionally charged issue. The red flag of patient confidentiality is often raised by providers, although their real fear is one of not knowing what purchasers and patients will do with provider-specific data. Purchasers do not need patient identifiers to manage successful UR programs, but without provider identification, the UR efforts cannot result in practice pattern changes. Provider fears are compounded by the poor quality of many hospital data sources, the potential legal action that could result from public disclosure of real—or perceived—poor performances, and the absence of accepted standards for medical practice that would facilitate meaningful comparisons of provider behavior.

This issue will be hotly debated in coming years. As more private purchasers sign contracts with peer review groups, two areas should be watched closely. Will hospitals cooperate and allow peer review groups access to private patient data? Will peer review groups release provider-specific profiles to private clients for their review and analysis?

The Peer Review Improvement Act of 1982 speaks to the first question by giving PROs access to the records for private-pay plans. However, fiscal intermediaries, UR firms, and others that do not receive PRO designation will not have automatic access and will need the support of local business and labor, especially those who serve as hospital trustees.

The second question is one that will challenge the physician leadership of peer review organizations and test their commitment to private review. If release of provider-specific data to private clients is inhibited, the enthusiasm of the purchaser community for peer review will be tempered. If, however, provider-specific profiles become a product that peer review groups sell in the marketplace, the purchaser community will be eager to do business. Striking a balance between the needs of the purchaser/consumer and the legitimate protection of the provider from damaging use of less than accurate data will be difficult.

One solution to the issue of access to data is the passage of state legislation that mandates disclosure of provider-specific information. In 1982 Iowa and Indiana passed just such bills. These measures—combined with private carriers' (e.g., the Blues in Arizona and Kansas City) acceptance of DRGs as a payment system for private patients and the growth of state all-payer payment systems symbolized by recently passed laws in Massachusetts and West Virginia—are other approaches being used to counter provider resistance to data access.

The interpretation of the Indiana law is being debated, and there has not yet been a resolution as to who will be responsible for its implementation or the degree to which physicians will control the release of information. The Iowa legislation mandates implementation of the uniform bill (UB–82) and creation of a statewide data clearinghouse to collect and disseminate provider-specific utilization and price information for all payers.

Case-Specific vs. System Cost Impact

UR critics, as well as supporters who insist on immediate results, can correctly point out that a dollar potentially saved by the identification of a patient who should no longer be in acute care is not a dollar saved in reality, unless the patient is actually sent elsewhere. And, not unlike the TV program "St. Elsewhere," there often is nowhere else to go. While not the fault of UR, the fact remains that in many cases the cost of the review itself is simply additive. It costs the same to identify a patient who should be transferred to a nursing home but for whom no openings exist as it does to identify one for whom the less expensive alternative care setting is available.

In addition, as the volume of services is better controlled by review strategies and as hospital occupancy rates begin to decrease, hospitals often increase their charges, thereby at least partially offsetting expected savings. UR programs in Minneapolis and Iowa have experienced this phenomenon. Both communities have, through alternative delivery systems and communitywide UR programs, reduced hospital utilization, yet charges have risen as hospital administrators spread their fixed costs over fewer patients. Savings will prove elusive in the absence of an equal commitment to controlling the hospital price side of the equation and to reducing excess capacity, whether through government action or market forces.

The willingness of companies such as Deere to stick with their UR programs is welcome evidence of growing employer sophistication and recognition that long-term solutions are dependent upon investment in short-term efforts like UR. Integrating utilization control with reimbursement changes and capacity controls is the essence of long-term cost-management strategies. A Deere representative summarized the company's position to Congress in 1980:

> Any effort to cost justify a review program without holding constant hospital "price" considerations is fallacious. The objectives of the PSRO and private review efforts are principally focused on monitoring quality of care and assuring that services are delivered in the most appropriate setting—whether that be inpatient, outpatient, or ambula-

tory. The review program should be held accountable only for achieving reductions in inpatient acute care services "volume," not reductions on the escalation of "price" levels charged by hospitals. As a private enterprise, we are of course, concerned that successful inpatient volume reductions may simply cause a corollary per unit price increase in aggregate expenditures for health care costs. However, hospital cost/pricing considerations fall outside the purview of our expectations of private review. The private sector, as well as the government, should manage the price per unit price or aggregate cost issue with the health care industry as a separate, albeit interrelated, issue to utilization review. (Heinze 1980)

Who Should Perform Utilization Review?

In effect, the 1982 federal legislation gives PROs a franchise with area limitations and at least the imprimatur of being certified as effective, since the government, as the nation's largest purchaser, has the most to lose from a weak system. For the first time, these UR organizations will be subject to tight performance standards. The comfort of the PSRO federal grant has been replaced by the rigors of PROs competing for federal contracts that will have termination provisions. Private purchasers will still be free to shop for review services, but any PRO that can establish its effectiveness will have a major marketing advantage due to its statutory access to private patient data and the ability to compare those data with the results of its Medicare review. Finally, hospitals and physicians, for all their objections to outside review requirements, will be more supportive of PROs being used by private payers rather than having medical record departments filled with competing and conflicting review groups, each demanding different information for different clients.

The Next Generation of Utilization Review

The 1970s may be described as the first generation of UR, the period of trial and error in the development of a national system. The second generation begins with the advent of private purchaser support and Medicare moving to a case-mix system in which utilization and reimbursement are related to each other. The effects of these changes will dominate most of the 1980s. What lies ahead?

Efficiency and efficacy in medical intervention will be rewarded. The marketplace is moving away from cost-based reimbursement. Purchaser demands for accountability are intensifying, and competition for patients is increasing. UR, as a mechanism to profile provider utilization patterns and communicate with physicians over identified problem areas, has become a critical element of this new era. The challenge is clear: quality health care at affordable costs. Given all the pressure for alternative delivery systems and regulatory approaches such as rate setting, UR systems may soon be seen as one of the few remaining defenses for fee-for-service medicine. Employers can also generally be said to support the continuation of the fee-for-service system, at least as one of the options in an era of increasing choice.

By the late 1980s, trends suggest that virtually all major private purchasers will have UR programs tied directly to reimbursement, and that purchasers will increasingly use UR data in negotiations with providers. Review will probably have graduated from its acute inpatient care focus to cover care in ambulatory facilities, hospices, homes, and physicians' offices. It also seems likely that the current, very real, constraints posed by the difficulty of linking physician and hospital records, especially for outpatient care, will be overcome.

Perhaps the most dramatic and challenging long-range implication emerging from the UR movement is the development of national standards of medical practice. Despite the predictable objections to "cookbook medicine" and interference with the physician's decision-making prerogatives, the fact remains that the basic concepts of UR and provider accountability are predicated upon measures of performance that are not location-specific. While there is no intimation that all physicians should practice in a like manner, there is no medical excuse for the variation in practice patterns that now exists, and UR can be expected to narrow of the accepted range of variations. Providers whose practice patterns fall outside the range will be subject to scrutiny and may face reduced reimbursement. The development of outcome-validated standards will be the next great advance toward a more uniformly high-quality, less wasteful, delivery system.

REFERENCES

Blumberg, M. S. "Regional Differences in Hospital Are Standardized by Reported Morbidity." Unpublished paper. Oakland, Calif.: Kaiser Foundation Health Plan, Inc., 1981.

Dixon, R. H., and J. Lazlo. "Utilization of Clinical Chemistry Services by Medical House Staff." Archives of Internal Medicine 134(1974): 1064–1067.

Glass, H. S. "Data for PSRO Objective Setting." Paper presented before the National Professional Standards Review Council, Washington, D.C., March 14, 1978.

Griner, P. R., and F. Liptzin. "Use of the Laboratory in a Teaching Hospital." Annals of Internal Medicine 75(August 1971):157–163.

Heinze, D. Testimony before the U.S. House of Representatives, Commerce and Energy Committee, July 1980.

Perrott, G. S. *The Federal Employers Health Benefits Program: Enrollment and Utilization of Health Services 1961–1968.* Washington, D.C.: Department of Health, Education, and Welfare, Health Services and Mental Health Administration, 1971.

Weisinger, R., K. J. Roghmann, J. W. Gavett, and S. M. Wells. "Inpatient Hospital Utilization in Three Prepaid Comprehensive Health Care Plans Compared with a Regular Blue Cross Plan."*Medical Care* 14(September 1976):721–732.

Wennberg, J. E., and A. Gittelsohn. "Variations in Medical Care Among Small Areas." *Scientific American* 246(April 1982):120–134.

5

Health Care Coalitions

Willis B. Goldbeck

INTRODUCTION

Large private employers spent the 1975–80 period awakening to the general cost-containment problem. Many became, to a large degree, supportive of the regulatory system that the federal government and the states were adopting. They also began to take the first, rather tentative, stabs at cost containment, through benefit design changes and increased demands for the data needed to compare the price and utilization patterns of providers. By 1980, major employers had learned that federal regulation alone was not the answer, nor could most insurers and providers be counted on to make significant changes to systems that were, from their perspective, successful. Further, they came to recognize that benefit design changes and other measures they could take as individual companies would not be of such magnitude as to have a significant impact on communitywide utilization, reimbursement, or system capacity, principally hospital beds and high-technology equipment.

Faced with these facts, and insurance premium increases that often exceeded 20 percent, employers came to realize cost management depended on the evolution of a strategy. A comprehensive strategy would have to integrate those cost-management activities that a company could undertake unilaterally and internally, such as benefit design changes, with those that the company could directly influence but which were external, such as hospital trustee education or contracts for utilization review. Finally, it became apparent that there remained major components of a strategy which could only be accomplished through collective action. Examples include alternative delivery system development, community health planning, multiple employer utilization review programs, community education programs, and the utilization/price data systems upon which to base other cost-management actions. Coalitions, or local business groups on health, are the institutional response to the growing awareness of the need for collective action.

As providers and insurers came to recognize the new seriousness on the part of employers, the expected happened. They tried to gain access and/or sought to initiate their own coalitions. Today, the American Medical Association (AMA), American Hospital Association (AHA), the Health Insurance Association of America (HIAA), and Blue Cross/Blue Shield Associations all have offices and programs designated to represent their interests in the coalition movement.

The next section discusses the various definitions of coalitions. It is followed by sections on the origins of coalitions; their characteristics and work agenda; examples of coalition accomplishments; and issues and trends relevant to the next generation of coalitions.

DEFINITIONS AND NUMBERS

Coalitions are associations with purchaser representation whose primary reason for being is to promote local rather than national health care cost-containment efforts. It is regional, state, county, city, or other nonnational geopolitical boundaries that define the scope of each group. Therefore, the Washington Business Group on Health, a national association of large employers, may in fact be a coalition of employers, or the AHA a coalition of hospitals, or the Dunlop Group (see next section) a coalition of association representatives. However, none of these is a coalition in the sense applicable to this discussion.

Furthermore, organizations with objectives other than medical care cost management are not considered to be coalitions. Thus, health systems agencies, trade organizations, professional associations, or their committees, are not coalitions, although they may be the catalyst for one, or even become one, through reorganization and the subordination of their mission to the primary goal of cost management.

There are two basic coalition models. There are coalitions that have, as equal members, most if not all of the major interests represented, in particular, both purchasers and providers. There are also those whose membership is limited to a specific interest (e.g., private sector employers) or a single but comprehensive category, such as purchasers, which may include government and labor.

The philosophical basis for each of these models is enlightening. The all-parties model is predicated upon the assumption that real change will occur only when all parties to that change work together. Furthermore, providers have a knowledge base that coalitions need to succeed and can help employers avoid either "reinventing the wheel" or taking actions that reflect misperceptions of the delivery system. In contrast, purchasers in the more restrictive coalition model start with the premise that they must, in the vernacular, get their act together without the pressures that result from having every interest represented at the table. They point out that, as purchasers, they are not invited to join the providers' coalitions, such as medical societies or hospital councils. The purchasers feel the need to set their own agenda and become armed with knowledge and data before they can approach the providers from a position of comparable strength.

It is important to recognize that nearly all of the purchaser-only coalitions fully understand the need to communicate with other interested parties. Most have established liaison systems, but they have adopted the position that formal membership is appropriately limited to those with the common interest and perspective of the purchaser.

There is no exact count of coalitions because of the absence of a universally accepted definition and of a source invested with the responsibility and resources to keep an ongoing tally. However, the growth of this phenomenon is easy to substantiate. Ten years ago, there were none that would fit today's description or purpose. By the mid-70s a handful were locally developed; between 1978 and 1981, the few had become approximately 50 as the concept had gained attention and the support of national organizations; and by early 1983 the total had doubled and a growth rate of roughly 25 per year was established. This growth is all the more impressive because most of it occurred in a period when the economy was in a recession and employers were reducing their commitments to outside organizations. The first organized effort to track coalition formation and programs was conducted by the U.S. Chamber of Commerce Clearinghouse on Business Coalitions for Health Action. The March 1983 edition of its directory lists 105 groups that meet three criteria: there must be significant representation by nonhealth businesses as purchasers of health care, the membership list must have been submitted to the Clearinghouse for documentation, and some sort of cost-containment strategy must have begun or be near implementation.

As informal review of emerging coalitions by the Washington Business Group on Health has identified at least 25 more that plan to initiate activities in 1984. In December 1983, the coalition office of the AHA published its first coalition directory. Based on the cooperative efforts of the AMA, HIAA, the Blues, AFL-CIO, and the Business Roundtable, the directory is a computerized record much like that of the Clearinghouse, though based on less specific criteria. It lists 123 groups.

In addition, specialized listings are beginning to emerge. For example, the Office of Health Promotion and Disease Prevention in the U.S. Department of Health and Human Services (DHHS) is nearing publication of a directory of the health promotion activities of coalitions it surveyed in 1983.

Currently, the rate of development far surpasses any existing tracking system. Leadership and staff change frequently, and the evolution of a group often has nebulous beginnings (e.g., an ad hoc committee of benefit managers). Although confusing for those who want to chronicle events, the rate and vitality of the movement's evolution is testimony to its seriousness and potential to cause change.

COALITION ORIGINS

Coalitions have a variety of origins: local business, local associations, health systems agencies (HSAs), insurers, national organizations, foundations, and government. Emerging from the growing realization of the need for a cost-management strategy that involves collective as well as unilateral action, coalitions have also served to meet the employer's need to become politically active at the state and local levels rather than depending only on national associations operating at the federal level. There is no limit to the number of groups that may develop. Increasingly, areas have more than one, as the multiparty and all-purchaser models learn to coexist. Networks of city and county groups are forming and working with their statewide counterparts. The stimulus comes from an increasing number of sources, and the potential agenda expands in proportion to the employer's growing sophistication and economic influence in a time of resource constraint. In general, the multiparty models are started by health care organizations and chambers of commerce, whereas purchaser groups are more likely to have been started by local businesses, labor, HSAs, and government in its role as catalyst or employer.

Local business

As with other initiatives, local leadership is frequently the most significant factor in determining whether or not an idea will lead to successful institutional development. Several of the coalitions are the result of the efforts of local business persons who felt an increasingly compelling need to take that next step in cost management: collective action. Examples include the San Diego Employer's Health Cost Coalition, the Fairfield-Westchester Business Group on Health, the Employers Health Care Coalition of Greater Los Angeles, and the Lehigh Valley Business Conference on Health.

Local associations

Frequently, a chamber of commerce health committee is a catalyst. Generally, these committees were started as part of the chamber's economic development program and were supportive of an expanding health care industry. Because the chamber retains the economic development responsibility as its primary function and may receive substantial financial support from its health industry members, it has often been better for the chamber to facilitate the formation of a separate coalition than to engage in the cost-management battle itself. The same can be said for other local industry associations.

Initiated by the Philadelphia Chamber of Commerce, PENJER-DEL (encompassing Philadelphia, southern New Jersey, and Delaware) is one of the oldest (1977) coalitions started by a local association. The New York Business Group on Health is an example of a coalition started in cooperation with, and initially housed by, a local chamber. Now in its third year, it has become totally independent. The Tidewater Health Coalition in Virginia resides organizationally in the Portsmouth chamber but serves a region of seven metropolitan areas. The Jefferson County Medical Society (a multiparty group in Birmingham, Alabama), the Arizona Association of Industries (purchaser-only group in Phoenix), and the Atlanta Chamber of Commerce (a multiparty group) are other examples of coalitions started by already existing local associations.

Health systems agencies

Rising interest in coalitions occurred simultaneously with the growth in employer support of health planning and the decrease in governmental support. Of the whole federally funded planning system, the local Health Systems Agencies (HSAs) were the component most vulnerable to budget cuts. However, many of them had a history of successful contact with industry, and it was natural that many HSA directors would consider building upon their industry relationships to develop coalitions. The HSAs had one major advantage: they were the repository of vitally needed data about the local health care system. They also had experienced staff and were a vehicle for local planning, which many employers already supported. However, all this was outweighed by negative feelings toward the HSA and/or government planning in general.

Employers, even at the national level, do not speak with one voice on issues such as planning. For example, the U.S. Chamber favored terminating federal support of local health planning, while the Washington Business Group on Health has urged the retention of a modified system. Several local coalitions became politically active in supporting planning at the federal level and also established new local mechanisms that attempted to fill the increasing void created by federal cutbacks.

In the past two years HSAs in Portland, Seattle, Vermont, and San Diego have provided the leadership for coalition formation and projects. The Portland coalition is multiparty, while those in Seattle and Vermont are purchaser-only. Of equal significance are coalitions that actively support local planning. For example, the Greater Cleveland Coalition on Health Care Cost Effectiveness (led by TRW) and industry-led efforts in North Carolina (Burlington Industries) and Virginia (Reynolds Metals) have resulted in state government support for new planning systems. In Iowa the HSA was instrumental in developing a successor organization, the Health Policy Corporation of Iowa.

Insurers

HIAA has sought to promote state rate-setting programs and has assisted in the development of coalitions that might in turn support rate setting. The most significant result of this effort was the Maryland Health Care Coalition, which has worked closely with the Maryland rate-setting and regulatory agencies and obtained the first review letter from the Department of Justice verifying that the coalition's agenda did not appear to violate antitrust statutes. HIAA has also been active in Illinois and Milwaukee, Wisconsin. By contrast, the Blues have been more active through their local plans than through an organized effort of the national association. In Oklahoma, for example, the Blues and the state chamber of commerce were the catalysts behind Governor Nigh's cost-containment conferences, which led to the creation of a coalition in Tulsa. The Blues also supported the development of the New York Business Group on Health and hosted the Philadelphia Area Committee on Health Care Costs and the Washington, D.C. area coalition.

National organizations

In the late 1970s, the Washington Business Group on Health began a program of technical assistance to local groups that wanted to start or become coalitions. The U.S. Chamber established a Health Action program, which called for increased collective activities at the local level. The AHA Voluntary Effort collected information on coalitions and promoted the multiparty model as having the greatest promise of success. The AMA's coalition office and corporate visitation program have urged employers to include physicians in coalitions.

In 1981 the Business Roundtable established its Health Initiative, a component of which is to encourage members to support local coalition activities. Also in 1981, Harvard professor John Dunlop organized a forum for representatives of the AMA, the Blues, HIAA, AHA, the AFL-CIO, and The Business Roundtable to discuss health care cost issues. This informal gathering has been mistakenly characterized as a coalition. The confusion arose because the first joint statement was in support of local coalition development and, both individually and collectively, these organizations encourage their members to paticipate in coalition activity.

Finally, the U.S. Chamber Foundation finances a coalition network known as the Clearinghouse on Business Coalitions for Health Action. It is staffed by the chamber and publishes a coalition directory and newsletter and holds periodic conferences under the leadership of a national advisory committee.

Foundations

The John A. Hartford Foundation has been the leader in supporting coalition efforts, having awarded multiyear grants to the Utah Health Cost Management Foundation and the South Florida Health Action Coalition. The Utah program has all parties involved and was organized as a result of a cost-management study performed by Lewin and Associates, Inc. for the Utah legislature. In South Florida, a purchaser-only coalition was started after Governor Graham urged major private employers to join him in a cost-management project. The developmental work was conducted jointly by the local Chamber and the Health Systems Agency. In both cases, Hartford grants facilitated the formation of a coalition for which considerable progress had already been made. Hartford has also provided funding to the New York Business Group on Health for a program to help small employers identify and assess health-related problems.

The Robert Wood Johnson Foundation, in conjunction with the AHA and Blue Cross/Blue Shield Association, has established a program that seeks to stimulate the development of new coalition projects. It is entitled Community Programs for Affordable Health Care, and through it the foundation plans to commit some $16 million in 1983–84 in grants to 10 to 20 coalitions. To be eligible, applicants must involve at least three of four major interest groups: hospitals, third-party payers (public or private), employers, and unions. However, the sponsoring organization may be an all-purchaser coalition, a hospital, or any other 501(c)(3) community organization. The stated principal goal is to develop a program, based on an analysis of the community's recent health care cost problems, to reduce significantly the future growth of health care expenditures in the community. In 1983, the first series of grants were awarded to support initiatives in San Diego, Erie (Pa.), Pittsburgh, Minneapolis, Worchester (Mass.), and Iowa.

CIGNA Corporation has announced a two-year program of support to local coalitions. The grants, of which eleven have been announced, ranging from $5,000 to $50,000, are for specific cost-management projects undertaken by coalitions and thus are not designed for coalition development as such. Priority consideration will be given to the creation and use of health cost data bases and to communication programs for health promotion and cost containment. Other projects, such as developing HMOs and preferred provider organizations, are also encouraged. To be eligible, a coalition must be able to match the CIGNA grant, be a 501(c)(3) corporation, and have an employer majority.

Government

Perceptions of cost shifting, resulting in part from government cutbacks and reduction of commitments to health planning and utilization review, have been a stimulus for coalition development. State government concerns about rising costs have also been a direct catalyst for the coalitions in Utah, Kentucky, Iowa, Florida, and Oklahoma. Increasingly, state and local governments are also participating in coalitions as employer/purchasers. In addition, DHHS has encouraged coalition development through the Bureau of Health Planning, three regional planning centers that it has funded, and the National Council on Planning and Development.

PROFILE

Considering the number of catalysts for coalition development, their varied composition, and their average age of less than three years, it is hardly surprising that they do not conform to an easily catalogued set of structures. Nonetheless, a profile of the coalitions that meet our definition does emerge.

Goal

The goal of most coalitions is the development of new mechanisms to reduce the rate of medical care cost escalation. For some, this entails only educational activities. For others, it means establishing the vehicle through which private purchasers can exercise collective economic clout. Some use coalitions for turf protection, and for still others coalitions are the means to immediate collective actions for achieving a single objective, such as the 1982 Massachusetts rate-setting law, which was the direct result of a multiparty coalition instigated by business and commercial insurance leaders.

Membership

As indicated, the multiparty groups have members drawn from both purchasers and providers. The purchaser groups may be business only or may include labor and/or government. Of the coalitions in the U.S. Chamber of Commerce Clearinghouse Directory, slightly over 50 percent are purchaser-only. Interestingly, the multiparty groups have a membership that averages 65 percent purchasers, and 12 have over 75 percent. The list compiled by the AHA's Voluntary Effort gives a different picture, because it includes local medical societies that have initiated cost-containment discussions with the business community. However, we would not construe such discussions as constituting a coalition.

Coalitions are not consumer groups in the sense of involving citizen participation, and in most cases consumers are not assigned designated slots on boards. Exceptions include the Kentucky Health Costs Coalition, in which 4 of the 34 members are consumer representatives, and the Arizona coalition, in which hundreds of small business and consumer groups participate.

Financing and staffing

Coalitions typically have low budgets; the average is under $50,000, and members' dues are the primary source of funds. Contributions by member companies to assist in start-up are also common. The few programs with large budgets include those in Utah and South Florida, which have grants from the John A. Hartford Foundation. Staffs are, in whole or in part, voluntary for nearly two-thirds of the coalitions, and fewer than 10 percent have more than three full-time paid staff. Coalition leaders are also becoming increasingly adept at obtaining in-kind services and shared programs. The trend is toward larger budgets and full-time staff, but there is also a strong desire to keep these groups small and use the membership, through task forces, for much of the work. Also, observers should not be misled by the common coalition practice of identifying staff as volunteers. In most cases, these people are not volunteers in the community sense; they are fully paid representatives of participating organizations, who feel that the use of their time is consistent with the objectives of their employer. Typical backgrounds of staff include experience with HSAs, insurance companies, PSROs, and benefits consulting firms.

Corporate structure

Some coalitions have chosen to remain unincorporated, and a few are incorporated as associations. However, the vast majority of those either already incorporated or in the application stage qualify under the 501(c)(3) tax exempt provisions of the IRS code. In interviews, it becomes apparent that many of the groups begun so tentatively just a year or two ago now view themselves as permanent.

Work agenda

The Chamber Clearinghouse survey that led to the directory identified five agenda topics: benefit design, data, alternative delivery systems, health education (including self-education about the cost issues), and health planning. However, that categorization omits two major items, trustee education and utilization review. Replies to the survey showed that data (for utilization and claims control) and health education were the most frequently mentioned agenda topics. More importantly, over 50 percent of the respondents indicated that all five topics were on their agenda, thus signifying the coalition as the place for multifaceted and integrated collective action. The development of good data on which to base benefit design changes, provider negotiations, and employee health education is the number one priority, according to interviews conducted by the Washington

Business Group on Health, the survey of the Business Roundtable Health Initiative, and surveys conducted by several consulting firms.

At this stage in the life of most coalitions, the agenda is more a reflection of interest and concern than of actual programs being implemented. This would be especially true for the alternative delivery system and health planning categories. It is of real significance that the coalition agendas parallel the needs that have been identified by both the public and private sectors as essential for lasting cost management. The coalitions' collective agendas represent an organized effort at seeking a balance between market forces and regulation.

ACCOMPLISHMENTS

The three most commonly asked questions about coalitions are: Are they just a fad? Are they successful? Are they the cause of adversarial relations between purchasers and providers?

Fad?

During the past three years, coalitions have grown in total numbers and membership size. They have become a presence on the state and local health care finance, planning, and delivery scene and have captured the attention of employers, government at all levels, insurers, providers, foundations, and labor. These years were not a period when corporate America was seeking new excuses to expend dwindling financial resources. Yet, the coalitions continue to grow, and virtually none have either closed or been reduced in size. The economic pressures have actually been helpful, forcing the companies to take more concerted action to manage medical expenditures. The companies now realize that collective action is a necessary component of a successful cost-management strategy. And, as in other movements, success breeds followers. The better recognized groups are besieged with surveys, visitors, and those who would like to emulate their efforts. In contrast, just five years ago, it took a major organizing effort to have business leaders agree to attend a meeting to consider the formation of a local coalition. Today, requests for assistance flow regularly, and groups are forming faster than anyone can accurately track. Finally, albeit sadly, the enormity of the medical care cost problems, accentuated by the anticipated Medicare deficit and premium increases reaching 40 percent, can make even the most marginally successful coalition seem like a wise investment. No, coalitions are not a fad.

Success?

As to whether or not they are successful, there is much more that we do not know than there are facts to report. Most coalitions are less than three years old. They are local and owe no pass/fail reports to anyone other than their members, and there are no common criteria upon which to base an evaluation. Therefore, we are left to assess the record of those few that have a history and the stated objectives of the others. If a coalition sets out to educate its members and does so while sustaining their support, then it could be deemed successful. Similarly, if the coalition establishes as a priority the development of a hospital comparative data system (PENJERDEL), or a multiemployer utilization review program (Minneapolis), or the development of special programs for small business (New York Business Group on Health), then the accomplishment of the objective can be rated a success even though one may have to wait for years to see if the hoped-for impact on the medical care market occurs.

Based on two measures, the coalition movement is already a success. First, more than 1,000 employers are now participating in one or more coalitions. Second, providers view their potential economic and political impact as too significant to ignore. Several examples demonstrate the diversity of coalition successes.

The Toledo Business Coalition on Health Care was formed in 1981 and immediately placed health planning at the top of its agenda. When the state defunded the HSA, the coalition created North-West Ohio Health Planning (NWOHP), Inc. In March 1983, the coalition and NWOHP successfully convinced the state of Ohio to reverse its certificate-of-need approval for a $25 million 97-bed expansion of a suburban hospital. This was the first time the state of Ohio had reversed a CON approval.

The Health Policy Corporation of Iowa (HPCI) was charged with implementing the recommendations of the Governor's Commission on Health Care Costs. Within a few months, HPCI has successfully generated legislation that passed the house and senate by overwhelming margins. The act created a new hospital and physician-specific utilization data reporting system, required a consumer majority on the Blue Cross/Blue Shield board, and ended anticompetitive restrictions on hospitals' rights to hire certain medical specialists.

The Health Care Committee of Cleveland Associated Industries is a coalition in a rural community of 30,000 northeast of Chattanooga, Tennessee, that has one private and one county hospital and 65 physicians. It represents an example of the educational role that a coalition can play and of the lasting commitment to orderly change that employers who work with coalitions have learned is necessary. The following description was provided by the chairman of the coalition, who is also chairman and chief executive officer of a local firm.

Cleveland Associated Industries was formed in 1962 "to use the talents and resources of industry for the betterment of the community."

The association has a $60,000 budget, one full-time employee, and 33 manufacturing members including Olin Corporation, M & M Mars Candy Company, Westvaco, Owens-Illinois, Bendix Corporation, Magic Chef, and American Uniform. Company representatives are only the top one or two executives on the local scene.

The Health Care Committee was formed in December 1977 to find ways to control the health care costs of member firms.

Most of the first year was spent researching the topic. HMOs and IPAs were explored. Meetings were held with the head of the Tennessee Hospital Association, local hospital administrators, doctors, insurance company representatives, and our own employees.

The second and third years were spent surveying members' health insurance plans, examining various cost-saving possibilities, recommending changes to the members, and then having members implement many of those changes. These include:

— working toward an 80/20, or even a 50/50, split with employees on estimated health care premiums

— using front-end deductibles for each hospital visit

— requiring second opinions on certain elective surgery

— encouraging the use of out-patient services and one-day surgery

— having a coordination for benefits clause

— extending the waiting period on preexisting conditions

— consideration of self-funding

— asking the insurance carrier for help in redesigning the health care plan to make it less costly

— educating employees on who really pays the medical bills (not the insurance company), etc.

We also decided that businessmen needed to get politically involved in the health care scene.

The fourth and fifth years have been devoted to making further changes in health care plans. For instance, four small companies banded together and self-funded. One company has a rebate plan wherein employees share in savings from underutilization of estimated health care costs (in 1981 $23,000 was rebated to 233 out of 306 employees in the plan). Other companies are pursuing wellness plans.

In summary, each company, through its top executive, has become much more involved in health care costs and has effected many cost-saving improvements.

The Midwest Business Group on Health can measure its impact on its eight-state region in several ways. Several new local coalitions have been started, and a program of user groups was created to convene employers who use the same insurance carriers so they could request a common data reporting system. Also, trustee education programs are having an impact on area hospitals. In conjunction with the Chicago Foundation for Medical Care and the Illinois Health Care Cost Coalition, the coalition stimulated the establishment of the Cook County Utilization Review Coordinating Council for private sector review. A ninth state, Nebraska, joined the coalition in 1983.

The New York Business Group on Health (NYBGH) in Manhattan has tackled a broad range of issues which, either directly or tangentially, have an impact on its members. It chaired the New York Self-Insurance Study Group, a project of the Governor's Health Advisory Council with staff support from the New York State's Health Planning Commission. The study involved a major survey of employers, analysis of recommendations for federal and state regulatory changes, and development of new self-insurance information services for private sector employers, a project the NYBGH will be undertaking. Also, it has promoted reform of state malpractice laws, working jointly with the New York Medical Liability Reform Coalition; it has developed emergency medical procedures for small business tenants of high-rise buildings; and it has conducted a project, funded by the John A. Hartford Foundation, to make small business aware of health cost issues and how to deal with them. In addition, NYBGH has reached agreement with Blue Cross/Blue Shield of Greater New York to develop hospital utilization reports. This will help individual employers and will also provide the coalition with an aggregate data base from which to formulate future cost-management priorities.

The Birmingham Employers' Coalition began in 1978. The following year, as a response to this all-purchaser organization, a new coalition, called the steering committee, was formed to bring together employers and physicians. Hospitals have been excluded, a position which the physicians endorse. The physicians have agreed to a major educational campaign to implement five recommendations. The usefulness and cost-effectiveness of routine admission batteries as related to hospital requirements and physician practice patterns are to be assessed. It is recommended that physicians admit only on an emergency basis on Friday or Saturday, and that concurrent review take place for all privately insured patients. To the extent that excess beds can be documented, actions are to be taken to remove such beds from the system, and movement is to be made towards the development of an indemnity method of payment of physician fees, replacing the current usual, customary, and reasonable (UCR) system.

The Employers' Coalition continued with its own agenda and developed a model health insurance package that encouraged preadmission testing, ambulatory surgery, and second opinions for surgery as well as the restructuring of coinsurance and deductible provisions. South Central Bell and other area employers have already adopted many of these provisions.

The Minnesota Coalition on Health Care Costs is a statewide, all-parties coalition. It was an outgrowth of the Minnesota Medical Association's study of health care costs, an effort that followed the example of the AMA-sponsored National Commission on Health Care Costs. Started in 1980, it had a self-imposed three-year sunset and thus has recently been forced to undergo a reassessment of its activities. Its members concluded that continuation for another three years was warranted. The coalition's mission statement is illustrative of the growth in sophistication and comprehensiveness that marks the leading groups.

The Goals and Strategies to fulfill this mission are:

1. To bring and keep together an interorganizational alliance that can jointly accomplish improvement in health and health care costs.

2. To encourage positive incentive-oriented changes and cost savings in health care delivery.

    a) To reduce the inappropriate demand for health care services, through changes in benefit structures and reimbursement policies that promote cost sensitivity for both providers and consumers and

    (1) Encourage and promote a plurality of competitive health care plans and practices.

    (2) Promote price and information disclosure to facilitate exercise of cost-effective choice.

    (3) Promote restructured benefit policies that reward cost-effective behavior.

    b) To identify and eliminate barriers to a free market approach to health care delivery.

    (1) Monitor current health legislation and recommend appropriate community response.

    (2) Identify existing legal and programmatic barriers for community action.

    (3) Communicate with business leaders, opinion makers, legislators, consumer organizations to influence policies and practices affecting health care economics and quality.

3. To monitor trends in health service prices and facilitate evaluation of the economic and quality impact of changes in health policy and alternative delivery forms.

4. To educate consumers (including the business community and governmental units), through existing and new community and business channels, in areas of:

   a) Availability and details of alternative forms of health care financing and health care practices.

   b) Health promotion activities and opportunities.

5. To educate providers in practice styles which are conservative of resources, without compromising the desired health outcome.

   a) To support effective quality and price surveillance and utilization review in all delivery plans.

   b) To encourage research in outcome evaluation techniques.

6. To respond to new issues and opportunities that affect the health and health care environment in Minnesota.

The Dayton Health Care Coalition, led by Mead Corporation, was started explicitly to increase competition in the Dayton medical marketplace. The coalition's efforts have resulted in the establishment of two HMOs. By 1982, approximately two-thirds of Mead's eligible employees had enrolled in the HMOs.

Adversarial?

Trends and interviews with employers suggest that, in the next two to five years, a majority of coalitions will begin as purchaser organizations and subsequently establish liaisons with their counterparts in the other interest groups. Multiparty groups will also grow, but at a slower rate, and, increasingly, purchaser groups will join with other constituencies to form alliances for targeted cost-management efforts that dissolve once the designated task is accomplished.

One such example is in Massachusetts, where the Massachusetts Business Roundtable led an effort to pass state all-payer rate-setting legislation that is designed to reduce, over a several year period, the traditional cost shifting by hospitals, which claim that Medicare pays less than its full share. Further, due in no small measure to the leadership of some of the commercial insurance carriers, the hospital discounts received by Blue Cross/Blue Shield will also be reduced, thus making a more competitive insurance market. The employers worked to obtain the support of labor, the Massachusetts Hospital Association, physicians, and the state. Key to the project's success was the granting of a Medicare waiver by the federal Health

Care Financing Administration. To aid in this process, which had to be accomplished in a very short time, the Massachusetts coalition received support from such national groups as the Washington Business Group on Health, thus establishing a model for local/national employer organization cooperation.

Examples demonstrating that relations can become adversarial as economic nerve centers are touched include the efforts of the Midwest Business Group on Health (private utilization review) and coalitions in Philadelphia (comparative data systems and increased ambulatory surgery facilities), Toledo (halting hospital expansion), and Michigan (bed-reduction programs). Adversarial relationships are often described as a negative feature, and one to be avoided. However, many in the business community view this as an intrinsic part of the process of reordering the priorities and incentives of the health care system.

In most cases thus far, the activity that initially had been adversarial led to a rapprochement of providers and purchasers. The evolution of the Michigan coalition into a multiparty model is a prime example. Increased competitive pressures, a surplus of physicians, and cost-containment pressures from federal and state governments make some local conflicts unavoidable. For some, this exemplifies what is wrong with coalitions; for others it is a symbol of why coalitions are needed and will have an increasing impact on local medical care markets.

THE NEXT GENERATION

To date, some 40 states and the District of Columbia have at least one coalition. Twelve states have four or more groups. Although no state has had an organized effort leading to the formalization of contact among coalitions, there are positive signs that the next generation of coalition activities will involve intra- and interstate networks and increasingly coordinated national policy projects.

Networks

California illustrates the evolution of networks within a single state. In California, coalitions, especially purchaser-only ones, are expanding along county lines to conform to the geographic areas of the county medical societies. There are eleven coalitions, ten of which are purchaser models, and three of which include government representation. The membership of the California chamber's statewide group is 70 percent business and 30 percent provider. The network concept has advanced beyond the simple exchange of information to include regular meetings of staff and members. Of special interest is the coordination of their responses to state legislative and regulatory initiatives.

Similar activity is occurring in South Carolina and North Carolina. Efforts to create networks are also underway in Pennsylvania, Tennessee, Florida, and New York. In Iowa, there is now a statewide multiparty group (Health Policy Corporation of Iowa), a statewide business and labor group, and seven local groups, six of which are purchaser-only models.

The Midwest Business Group on Health is the strongest example of a multistate program. One of its priorities is the establishment of local groups in its eight-state area. In addition, more informal meetings of groups from the same region will be increasingly common, as is already the case in Vermont, New Hampshire, Maine, and parts of Massachusetts.

National Policy Projects

Quite appropriately, most coalitions have focused their attention on local programs and state policy. Increasingly, concern over federal legislation and regulations, and the fact that most leading coalition members are national corporations, have given impetus to participation in national policy projects. For example, the Midwest Business Group on Health has made utilization review a high priority. To further its objective, it has joined with the Washington Business Group on Health to create a joint task force which, working with the American Medical Peer Review Association, has assisted Senate and administration staff on the design of the new professional review organization program.

The interests of employers in preserving a federal health planning program were expressed at the national level through several coalitions, such as the Northeast Indiana Business Group on Health, the Central Iowa Health Association, the Michigan Health Economic Coalition, the Toledo Business Coalition on Health Care, the Pittsburgh Business Group on Health, and the North Carolina Foundation for Health Planning. In early 1983, more than 20 coalitions joined with the Washington Business Group on Health in presenting to Congress their opposition to the weakening of the Federal Trade Commission's authority over the business and commercial practices of medical professionals.

Purchaser or Multiparty Model

In the next generation of coalitions, the lines between the two primary models are likely to blur. Within some communities, one model that is likely to emerge will combine a multiparty coalition, a purchaser (business) group, and joint projects. The purchaser groups will be much like the local medical society or hospital council in that they will exhibit a clarity of purpose and membership as well as the freedom to adopt unhomogenized policy positions. Purchasers will also be represented in the multiparty coalitions. Finally, specific projects or issues will result in the formation of temporary coalitions of groups that agree upon a single common objective.

ISSUES

Any movement that deals with a topic as complex and volatile as health care will raise some perplexing issues. Seven such issues for the coalition movement are: antitrust status; impact on quality of care; support or rejection by labor; access to institution- and physician-specific utilization data; impact on availability of care for the poor; price differentials among purchasers; and targets of opportunity.

Antitrust Status

Coalitions have come into existence to change the status quo in health care economics. If they are successful, not every individual or institutional provider will receive the same share of the economic pie as would otherwise be the case. Many people are therefore worried about the potential antitrust implications of some of the cost-management actions of coalitions. Especially for major employers, who are always sensitive to the risk of antitrust charges (regardless of merit), the prospect of joining forces with other purchasers, much less with both buyers and sellers, to rearrange the economics of an industry raises real concerns. Some groups have virtually ignored antitrust issues, while others have lawyers present at every meeting. Some fear that any concerted action to select the most cost-efficient providers will cause those excluded to bring suit; others fear that the law will prevent the establishment of price schedules; still others feel that there is nothing to fear, since their particular coalition is an educational and advisory group rather than an instrument of implementation.

There is no case law that clearly defines the antitrust ramifications of coalition activities. To assist coalition participants to minimize antitrust risk, the John A. Hartford Foundation funded the National Health Policy Forum to produce an antitrust guide, written by health lawyers Robert Halper and John Miles. Previously, lawyers John B. Reiss and Phillip A. Proger authored a discussion guide on the subject.

Both of those analyses reached essentially the same conclusions. Since there is nothing about coalition activity that is unique from an antitrust perspective, one can be reasonably guided by the existing body of antitrust procedure and interpretation. It was pointed out that the all-purchaser model is least vulnerable to antitrust actions, because it avoids having buyer and seller together. However, no model is risk-free, nor is any model a per se violation. Risk is increased when some members of a specific class (e.g., certain hospitals) are excluded from a coalition in which other members participate. Besides avoiding the obvious—such as fixing prices, engaging in boycotts, or creating monopolies—coalitions can minimize their risk by being the source of information upon which their members act, rather than acting for the members. As the Halper and Miles guidebook makes clear, the thrust of all analysis to date is simply that common sense and avoidance of clear violation will generally be adequate protection.

Quality of Care

The coalition movement is paralleled by the worksite wellness movement. Employers are increasingly aware of the value of healthy workers, and there is no indication that employers are seeking cheap medicine at the expense of employee health. Although a few employers may behave irresponsibly, there are direct financial/productivity and employee relation incentives for employers to ensure that employees receive appropriate medical care.

Coalition cost-management strategies increasingly focus on activities that reduce waste, abuse, and inappropriate utilization, including restructuring economic incentives and improving the regulatory framework, and analyzing utilization data to redesign benefits, develop wellness programs, and guide patients to the most appropriate care setting.

The coalition movement is not only a response to these strategies as espoused by individual purchasers but also a catalyst for them. The process will give new meaning to the old bromide "freedom of choice." Economic incentives that promote early discharge from the hospital and treatment in appropriate ambulatory settings ideally both are cost-effective and reduce the risk of nosocomial infections and other iatrogenic illness. In simple terms, one consequence of coalition activity may ultimately be the presence of increasingly informed purchasers negotiating with competing providers for the most appropriate balance of efficiency and effectiveness.

Labor Participation

The early period of coalition development witnessed little labor involvement. Of the groups formed before 1980, only six had labor involvement—1980 and 1981 saw only four more. However, nine of the groups formed in 1982 had labor members. Also, many of the groups, such as the Pittsburgh Business Group on Health, have had a formal labor liaison process from the start.

The absence of union participation in many of the coalitions should not be interpreted as a lack of interest in the health care cost issues or in coalitions themselves. At the national level, labor has a much longer history of concern for health policy and medical care costs than does business. That interest has not diminished. The AFL-CIO participates with the Dunlop Group and has endorsed its coalition statement in which each national organization pledged to encourage and assist its local members in coalition development. Other unions, such as the Service Workers, Steel Workers, and the United Auto Workers participate in coalition activity, and there are indications that the level of activity is on the rise. Also, numbers can be misleading. In many communities, there are several business leaders but only one or two labor leaders. For example, in Iowa, for business to be adequately represented on the state-level Business and Labor Coalition and the Health Policy Corporation of Iowa, Deere, Pioneer Hi-Bred, Rockwell International, Meredith Publishing, and Caterpillar are just a few of the firms that must be involved. Labor can be represented by a single representative of the AFL-CIO.

Access to Data

For a majority of the coalitions, developing a health services utilization data base is the top priority in order to meet many of their objectives. It is needed for negotiating preferred provider contracts that are based on an understanding of provider practice patterns and for designing wellness programs targeted to conditions that represent the greatest risks or generate the highest utilization. It is also necessary for redesigning benefits with cost-sharing and appropriateness incentives, such as ambulatory surgery and hospice, targeted to the actual and projected experience of the employees and dependents. Such a data base will also help target the curriculum of trustee education programs, identify excess bed capacity, and conduct utilization review. Many employers are requesting data through coalitions.

Coalitions have become an important vehicle enabling employers to gain access to utilization data. The most obvious reason is that it is more difficult for a hospital to refuse a request from a collection of the community's leading employers than from a single employer. However, even the hospital benefits from the coalition approach. Instead of ultimately having to deal with an array of requests from many employers, each of whom wants something a little different, the hospital can provide the coalition with a single data report and leave the company-specific analysis up to the coalition and its members. In turn, the fact that a significant number of employers are gathering the same data contributes to communitywide cost management to a far greater extent than would any number of employer actions taken independently.

Impact on Low Income Populations

The growth of coalitions, with their emphasis on cost management and shrinkage of the delivery system, has come at a time when government at all levels faces resource constraints impacting on commitment to health programs. Understandably, concern has been expressed for the potentially negative impact of coalition activities on those who have neither large purchasers to represent them nor insurance coverage. Of particular note is the possibility that forceful actions by a handful of large employers will cause providers who face tougher revenue constraints to reduce the level of services provided to those who cannot afford to pay. Few, if any, coalitions had care for the poor on their initial agendas. Furthermore, the admittedly inefficient hospital that a coalition seeks to close may be the very institution that provides needed care for the poor.

However, participation in coalitions has increased employers' awareness of the interdependencies between public programs and private sector initiatives. Employers who previously paid little attention to Medicare or Medicaid now do so regularly. At the local level, access issues, the future of public general hospitals, and the needs of teaching hospitals have become increasingly important topics at coalition meetings. Although there is no guarantee that all coalition activities will be sufficiently sensitive to the needs of the poor, the poor also stand to benefit from an informed private sector that is committed to an efficient and affordable delivery system.

Price Differentials

The employer community is being divided by the issue of all-payer vs. price differential systems. Those firms that benefit from Blue Cross discounts or believe they can successfully negotiate directly with providers usually oppose the all-payer approach that is favored by many commercial carriers, their clients, and many small employers who lack market strength. This issue has surfaced in Pennsylvania and Illinois, where the legislatures are considering rate-setting bills. In both cases, employers are divided on the issue.

Targets of Opportunity

Looking ahead, it is possible to foresee several areas that represent major future targets of opportunity for coalition action. These fall into two primary categories: legislation and cost management.

We predict that state-level legislative priorities will include bills to guarantee purchasers access to hospital- and physician-specific utilization data and price information, and the establishment of malpractice arbitration systems. State rate-setting systems will probably be proposed, some of which will be all-payer, while others will foster a more competitive approach. Also likely are the repeal of provisions in state medical practice acts that impede cost-efficient care delivery, and participation in the development of innovative Medicaid and other state long-term care systems.

For cost management, the opportunities are without limit. The potential areas of focus include negotiated provider arrangements based upon utilization and price comparisons; coordinated benefit design changes to establish second-opinion, ambulatory surgery, and prior approval programs that target the same procedures; and development of consumer information systems based on utilization data for the direct use of enrollees. Other important needs to be addressed include support of alternative delivery system development, communitywide consumer health education and cost awareness programs, and state and local capital needs assessment.

CONCLUSION

Coalitions are exciting because they represent a significant step forward in the evolution of cost management strategies at the employer and community levels. In the long run, the greatest contribution of coalitions may be that they provide an institutional base for cost-management activities. At the very least, coalitions are a symptom of the severity of the cost escalation problem and the seriousness of many, in communities of all sizes, to grapple with economically and ethically difficult issues. At their best, coalitions are the vehicle through which, in varying ways reflecting local conditions, all parties participate in moving our country closer to the dream of affordable care that is of high quality and accessible to all. Coalitions are not the only answer. However, despite the short duration of their existence, it is hard to imagine real progress being made without some comparable mechanism.

APPENDIX: SOURCES OF INFORMATION

Review of Secondary Data Sources

Independent resources for the study of coalitions as a private sector initiative in health care cost management are scant. There is no academic literature to review. Longitudinal evaluations have not been conducted. Many of the references discuss coalitions within a more comprehensive examination of business (employer/purchaser) involvement in health. Others are the result of specific constituencies (planner, physicians, hospitals, insurers, business) that have received, often through speeches, workshops, and conference papers, anecdotal information about coalitions, and guidelines for future involvement with coalitions.

National media coverage about coalitions has not been extensive. Some mention has been made in most of the business press (*Fortune, Business Week*, the *Wall Street Journal*) and some of the major newspapers such as the *New York Times* and the *Chicago Tribune*. Attention of the health press (the *New England Journal of Medicine*, newsletters, *Business Insurance Magazine*) has been growing but remains irregular. Association and health industry magazines cover coalition development with a general theme that can be characterized as one of warning their constituents that coalitions may become serious enough to warrant their attention and involvement.

Local media coverage, especially when a coalition is in its formative stage, has been extensive. Editorials are common, and all three television networks often cover the conferences that typically are part of the establishment of a coalition. Several coalitions have made a point of having a major media employer as a member. Others have worked closely with local reporters to expand the extent of health care coverage.

The best publicly available secondary sources for statistics are the directories published by the U.S. Chamber's Clearinghouse and the AHA. The directories are based upon periodic surveys of the coalitions and include information on membership, agenda, corporate structure and financing. As with all directories in a rapidly evolving field, no edition is current for very long. However, the staff of both organizations do try to provide supplements, and the National Advisory Committee is aware of most new coalition development. The Clearinghouse limits its coverage to those coalitions that have significant business participation.

The Washington Business Group on Health keeps files on coalitions for the use of its own members and for the work its staff does with coalitions. The HIAA has staff assigned to each of the coalitions with which it is involved. The AMA is the best source for information about medical society involvement. The American Health Planning Association publishes a newsletter covering planning agency participation in coalition development and coalition activities that relate to health planning.

Other Information

In preparing this book, the principal information sources were personal contacts within individual coalitions, materials provided by the coalitions, and the Clearinghouse Directory. Sources of available information are given below, although the lists are not exhaustive.

Organizations

Clearinghouse on Business Coalitions for Health Action. U.S. Chamber of Commerce, Washington, D.C.

The Business Roundtable Health Initiative. New York, N.Y.

Community Program for Affordable Health Care, Robert Wood Johnson Project. Chicago, Illinois.

The Washington Business Group on Health. Washington, D.C.

The American Medical Association (AMA), Office of Coalition Development. Chicago, Illinois.

The American Hospital Association. Chicago, Illinois.

The Centers for Health Planning:

  — The Western Center. San Francisco.

  — The Alpha Center. Bethesda, Maryland.

  — The Midwest Institute. Chicago, Illinois.

Health Insurance Association of America. New York, N.Y.

The American Health Planning Association. Washington, D.C.

Examples of coalition products

Group Health Association of America
Guide for Group Practice HMO, to Business/Health Coalitions. 1982

Kentucky Healthcare Coalition, Inc.
Kentucky Employers Handbook on Health Insurance Management Strategies. 1984

Maryland Health Care Coalition
Health Management, A Guide to Improve the Health of Your Employees. 1983

Midwest Business Group on Health
Newsletter

Minnesota Coalition on Health Care Costs
A Coalition Perspective: New Directions for Health Care in Minnesota. 1981

Gives the history, mission, and plans for the Minnesota Coalition's work in health planning, new market forces, and education.

Update Report
Newsletter

New York Business Group on Health
Newsletter
Self-Insurance and Health Care Benefits in New York State. 1983

PENJERDEL (Philadelphia)
Cost Effective Management of Health Benefit Programs. 1980

Philadelphia Area Committee on Health Care Costs
Something is Being Done About Rising Health Care Costs. 1979

Describes the progress made on the coalition's objectives concerning increased use of ambulatory surgery, reduction of unnecessary beds, and physician education.

South Florida Health Action Coalition
Benefits Design and Administration Guidelines. 1981

A reference tool for the review and modification of existing health benefits to contain rising costs based upon an inventory of the plan design and benefit administration strategies.

Business Industry and Health.

Newsletter

Utah Health Cost-Management Coalition

A Market Approach to Controls of Rising Health Care Costs. 1981

A basic primer advocating market forces as the essential element for long-term cost management.

The newsletters are available to the public.

Annotated bibliography

American Medical Association. *The Formation of Medicine/Business Coalitions.* Chicago: AMA, 1981.

A manual for local medical societies, giving the AMA perspective on coalitions with guidelines for involvement.

Bureau of Health Planning. *A Resource Guide for Securing an Increased Private Sector Participation in Health Planning.* Washington, D.C.: DHHS, 1981.

Guidelines for and examples of health systems agencies' involvement with coalitions.

"Business and Health." *Review* 14(November/December 1981).

A collection of articles by and about employers' involvement in health, with a focus on coalitions.

Goldbeck, Willis B., Richard Egdahl, and Diana Chapman Walsh, eds. *A Business Perspective on Industry and Health Care.* New York: Springer-Verlag, 1978.

The volume of the Springer series that provides a background for the development of the coalition movement.

Caulfield, Stephen, and Pamela Haynes. *A Report on Coalitions to Contain Medical Care Costs.* Washington, D.C.: Government Research Corporation, 1979.

One of the first papers to look at coalition development and attempt to organize the elements essential for success.

Coalitions for Health Care. A statement by the Dunlop Group, January 1982.

A joint statement in support of local coalition development signed by and available from AMA, AHA, Blue Cross/Blue Shield Association, HIAA, AFL-CIO, and the Business Roundtable.

"Controlling Health Care Costs: The Coalition Approach." *Medicine and Health: Perspectives* 35(25)June 22, 1981.

A brief review of coalitions as one part of the changing politics of health care.

Earle, Paul *The Voluntary Effort Quarterly*. December 1981.

An assessment of the state of coalition development and a listing of the 79 organizations which the VE staff defined as coalitions.

Ferman, John, and Allen Toon. "Employers Step Into the Jungle of Health Costs." *Insight* (March 1982).

A review of coalition development with a focus on nine California coalitions and their increasing impact on California hospitals.

Friedman, W. Robert. *Business Coalitions*. San Francisco: Montgomery Securities, 1982.

A leading financial analyst looks at the potential impact of business coalitions and concludes that the health care industry cannot afford to ignore the coalition movement.

Gartner, Michael. *Business Efforts to Influence Local Health Systems*.

Speech to an InterStudy Conference on Coalitions. Excelsior, Minn., InterStudy, 1981. (A clear statement and analysis of why and how a local business leader became a coalition activist.)

Halper, H. Robert, and John J. Miles. *An Antitrust Guide for Health Care Coalitions*. Washington, D.C.: National Health Policy Forum, 1983.

Health Action: Strategies to Improve Health and Contain Costs. Washington, D.C.: U.S. Chamber of Commerce, 1979.

Five volumes of guidelines and examples for health care cost management. These predate most coalitions but are frequently used by coalitions.

Iglehart, John K. "Health Care and American Business." *New England Journal of Medicine* 306(January 14, 1982): 120–124.

An excellent review of business involvement since the early 1970s placing the coalition initiative within that larger context.

Jaeger, Jon B., ed. *Private Sector Coalition: A Fourth Party in Health Care?* Durham, N.C.: Duke University Department of Health Administration, 1983.

Proceedings of a conference with papers presented by one business person (Chris York of Citicorp), several providers and consultants.

Lanning, Joyce A. *Coalition for Health Care: Theory and Practice*. Doctoral dissertation, University of Alabama at Birmingham, 1983.

The most current review of the literature. Examines the coalition movement from the perspective of interorganizational theory. Request copies from author.

Los Angeles County Medical Association. "A Colloquium on the Los Angeles Health Care Coalition." *LACMA Physician* (June 20, 1983).

A discussion with coalition chairman Arnold Glassman of ARCO and two physician participants.

The National Council for Health Planning and Resource Development. *Proceedings of Meeting on Coalitions for Local Health Planning and Antitrust Issues in Coalition Building*. Washington, D.C.: DHHS, 1981.

A compilation of presentations by Willis Goldbeck, Jan Ozga, Robert Halper, David Benor, and Michael Pollard.

Proceedings of the First Conference of the Clearinghouse on Business Coalitions for Health Action. Washington, D.C.: U.S. Chamber of Commerce, 1982.

Reiss, John, and Philip Proger. *Issues Concerning Antitrust Liability of Health Care Coalitions*. Washington, D.C.: Baker and Hostetler, 1982.

A discussion of court cases that provide guidance to coalitions concerned that their activities may make them vulnerable to antitrust charges. The respective roles of the Federal Trade Commission and Justice Department are described, and guidelines are provided for understanding the many different coalition functions that might be subject to antitrust action. The authors conclude that coalitions can organize their functions and projects with reasonable assurance that they will not violate antitrust laws.

Waldholz, Michael. "Businesses are Forming Coalitions to Curb Rise in Health Care Costs." *Wall Street Journal* (June 17, 1982).

Examples of coalitions, their reasons for coming into existence, and the reactions of the provider community to their presence.

6

Worksite Wellness

Anne K. Kiefhaber and
Willis B. Goldbeck

INTRODUCTION

The United States is experiencing a cultural shift. The long-held view that health is merely the absence of disease and can be restored through high-technology medical care is being tempered by the perception of opportunities to improve health status through environmental safety and altered personal lifestyles. The shift is reflected in a Louis Harris survey, which reported that 92.5 percent of those polled agreed with the statement:

> If Americans lived healthier lives, ate more nutritious food, smoked less, maintained proper weight, and exercised regularly, it would do more to improve our health than anything doctors and medicine could do for us.

A new word has been coined that summarizes the attempt to achieve optimal health: wellness. Programs that promote wellness include the identification and treatment of diseases or biological risks that lead to disease, such as hypertension and diabetes; behavior change, such as improved nutrition, physical fitness, weight reduction, and stress management; environmental changes that reduce exposure to hazardous or toxic substances or intolerable levels of stress; and educational efforts to increase awareness of the opportunities for self-improvement and the appropriate use of medical services.

Wellness activities can be observed in many aspects of American society. Wellness-related products—such as running apparel, vitamins, and biofeedback equipment—have become more than a $30 billion a year industry (Time, Nov. 2, 1981, p. 103). Food products are changing to meet consumer demands for more fiber and natural nutrients and less salt, caffeine, calories, and refined sugar. Advertising campaigns increasingly stress society's positive perception of wellness. Information about wellness is reaching the public through television, magazines, and best-selling books.

Several dominant themes account for the societal and, hence, workplace shift toward wellness. The nature of illness has changed during this century from acute infectious disease to chronic, lifestyle-related disease over which individuals have greater control. Today, three causes of death account for 71 percent of all deaths in the United States: cardiovascular disease (40.7 percent), cancer (23.9 percent), and accidents (6.7 percent) (National Center for Health Statistics 1983). Although the exact cause of the first two illnesses is still unknown, there are, clearly, predisposing risk factors, including high cholesterol, hypertension, obesity, diabetes, smoking, stress, exposure to toxic substances, and lack of exercise.

In addition, the relationship between lifestyle and incidence of illness has been more firmly demonstrated. For example, Dr. Lester Breslow at UCLA conducted a study to estimate the health effects of the following lifestyle practices: three meals a day, no snacks, breakfast every day, moderate exercise two or three times a week, seven or eight hours of sleep per night, no smoking, moderate weight, and moderate alcohol consumption. After following 7,000 persons for several years, the study concluded that the average 45-year-old male who observed zero to three of the above practices had a life expectancy of an additional 21.6 years, while the same person who followed six or seven of the rules could expect to live another 33.1 years—11.5 years longer (summarized in Cunningham 1982; for examples of other reports of studies demonstrating the effect of lifestyle, see Dawber 1980 and Bauer 1980).

For a variety of reasons, the worksite is a logical setting for wellness programs. Illness generates expenses for health insurance, workers' compensation, reduced productivity, absenteeism, and turnover. Statistics have been assembled that suggest how expensive ill health and risk factors are for employers. For example, one smoking employee is estimated to cost employers between $624 and $4,611 dollars annually more than a nonsmoking employee in medical costs, absenteeism, replacement costs, maintenance, property damage, other insurance increases, and lowered productivity (Kristein 1980, Weis 1981). Annually, more than 26 million work days are lost due to cardiovascular disease and hypertension (National Heart, Lung, and Blood Institute 1981), and some $19 billion in work loss days was attributed to excessive drinking in 1979 (Cunningham 1982).

Seen more positively, the worksite offers opportunities to facilitate healthy behavior. Most people spend one-third of their time at work. Workplace programs usually have higher participation rates than community programs. For example, New York Telephone achieved 90 percent participation in a multiphasic screening program, while a similar community program achieved a 30 percent participation rate, even with extensive publicity. In addition, the corporate culture can contribute positively or negatively to health-related behavior.

For some industries, the motivation to be current with societal trends comes from their product line. Wellness relates directly to the business of hospitals, drug and vitamin companies, device manufacturers, insurers, food producers, and fitness facility and equipment vendors. For others, incorporation of the concept can favorably affect advertising, recruitment, and public image.

This chapter first profiles worksite wellness programs. The organizations—such as hospitals, voluntary agencies, private firms, and insurance carriers—that market wellness services are then profiled. A discussion of the evidence regarding the effectiveness of these programs follows. Finally, some of the issues associated with the worksite wellness movement are discussed. Not within the purview of this chapter are the important areas of occupational health and safety, because they are separate programs and raise different issues.

PROFILE OF WORKSITE PROGRAMS

Most worksite wellness programs have developed piecemeal rather that through the implementation of a strategy. However, corporate strategies have emerged that integrate many aspects of work and health. Although still in the minority, companies such as General Dynamics have appointed committees to formulate health enhancement strategies that include representation from several departments, e.g., personnel, safety, medical, benefits, fitness, employee assistance, and corporate planning.

Statistical surveys of worksite wellness activities must be intrepreted with great caution. No survey has sought to sample every type of employer, nor has any survey recorded all of the elements of wellness programs. In addition, the geographic dispersion of worksite wellness makes pinpointing company efforts difficult. For example, a corporation may have an extensive program at a single location, such as its headquarters, that is reflected in a survey response, although there may be minimal activity at other locations. A consistent pattern does, however, emerge in surveys conducted by the Washington Business Group on Health in 1978 and 1982, the Health Research Institute in 1979 and 1981, and the benefits consulting firms of the Mercer Company and Towers, Perrin, Forster, and Crosby in 1982. Characteristics of that pattern include a rapid and sustained growth in the number of employers offering programs; integration with other elements of private sector cost-management initiatives; and reports of positive results, including employee satisfaction, reduced absenteeism and insurance costs, and modest measures of actual health enhancement.

Companies that have wellness programs do not necessarily make them available to all employees, and dependents or retirees may or may not be eligible to use them. IBM's program is available to all employees, retirees, and spouses at all locations, and the program at Xerox is available to all employees at all locations. Kimberly-Clark has a program for all employees, retirees, and spouses, but it is available at selected locations only, as is the Metropolitan Life program for all employees. New York Telephone has a wellness program for its high-risk employees, and Texaco has one for executives only.

One reason for the breadth and diversity of wellness programs is the large variety of individuals who design and conduct them. The first programs were predominantly initiated by very senior individuals within corporations who believed in the benefits of a corporate culture that promoted wellness. Now that wellness programs are becoming an accepted benefit, other departments are also initiating them. The motivation often reflects the source, i.e., cost when the program is started by the benefits department; morale and productivity when it is started by a human resources or industrial relations department; and health when it is started by the medical department. Corporate departments that have initiated wellness programs include: medical, benefits, human resources, training, personnel, safety, recreation, and special divisions established by senior management. Initiators have included doctors, nurses, health educators, trainers, social workers, psychologists, and people with backgrounds in physical fitness, marketing, personnel, and benefits.

Furthermore, the staff and facilities can either be worksite- or community-based. Many combinations occur. Kimberly-Clark has worksite wellness staff teaching courses on site, as do Pepsi, Northern Natural Gas, and Sentry Insurance. National ChemSearch also has its own worksite wellness staff but community facilities are used; at companies such as Rolm and IBM, on the other hand, community-based instructors (e.g., from private firms and the YMCA) use worksite facilities, and, in the case of IBM, community facilities as well. Some programs are run entirely by employee volunteers, as is the one at the Center for Disease Control, a part of the U.S. Public Health Service. At General Dynamics, employee volunteers work in conjunction with wellness program staff.

This section addresses the components that comprise a wellness strategy. There are many ways to group or describe wellness activities at the worksite. Figure 6.1 structures the descriptions of programs by arranging them in categories. The left side represents those that most overlap with medical care; the right hand side focuses more heavily on lifestyle changes. The categories are not presented as absolutes but rather as a set of organizing principles that can guide one through an exploration of worksite wellness.

→ Early detection of disease and biological risks reflect specific medical conditions that either represent illness or are potential biological precursors to illness. Examples include hypertension, diabetes, glaucoma, obesity, elevated cholesterol, and many forms of cancer. Program examples include hypertension screening, breast self-exam courses, and periodic physical examinations.

→ Control of disease and biological risk programs are designed to treat or control the illness identified by the above-mentioned screening programs. Most conditions in this category require medical intervention, which is most often provided through referral to community physicians and paid for by the company-sponsored insurance plans. Examples of programs that are commonly provided at the worksite include hypertension treatment, alcohol and drug abuse treatment, cardiac rehabilitation, and courses that help control obesity and cholesterol levels through diet changes.

→ Detection of high-risk behavior with known or suspected negative health consequences includes smoking, poor nutrition, inactivity, inappropriate reaction to stress, and weight above or below normal ranges. Health risk profiles, some computerized and others that can be self-scored, have been developed to help individuals determine the consequences of their risk behavior.

→ Methods to reduce high risk behavior include the provision of information, education, counseling, and incentives. For each risk behavior, there are a number of approaches. For example, to assist with smoking cessation, a company may provide several different educational programs, one-on-one counseling, a do-it-yourself program, and hypnosis.

The overall corporate culture can facilitate good health. Healthy behavior has a better chance of being sustained if it becomes the norm. Policies such as smoking restrictions, making time available for exercise and classes, helping individuals meet the demands of in-

FIGURE 6.1 Worksite wellness categorization

DISEASE & BIOLOGICAL RISK		HIGH-RISK BEHAVIOR		
Detection	*Control*	*Detection*	*Reduction*	*Corporate culture*
Hypertension screening	Hypertension control	Health risk appraisals	Information dissemination — seminars — literature — food labeling	Policies — smoking restrictions — flex-time — program eligibility
Glaucoma testing	Referral services for illness detected at the worksite	Health fairs		
Blood testing		Information dissemination about health risks	Classes	Management styles — environmental facilitation of healthy behavior — wellness programs
Diabetes screening			Self-help materials	
Cancer detection — breast self-exam — Hemoccult tests			Behavior modification	
Periodic physical exams			Incentives	
Weight assessments				

tegrating family with work through flex-time, job sharing, maternity and paternity leave, and part-time employment help to show the company's concern for the individual and its desire to promote healthy behavior. In addition, physical amenities—such as exercise facilities, the availability of nutritious food, a quiet room for relaxing, an attractive working environment, noise control, and day care centers—all promote good health.

Early Detection of Disease and Biological Risk

As more has been learned about the relationship between life-style and illness and as diagnostic technology has become available, the worksite has increasingly become the locus of detection and treatment programs. Medical screening programs that are designed to detect disease and/or biological risks include pre-employment physicals, periodic physicals, executive physicals, screens that target a particular risk or disease such as hypertension or glaucoma, and self-screening programs such as breast or testicle self-examination. These tests are conducted in a variety of ways, including on-site with company medical personnel and equipment; on-site through mobile screening units, community volunteers, or paid personnel; and off-site but paid for by the company.

Support for these physical exams stemmed from the belief that many diseases and biological risk factors could be successfully controlled if caught early. This theory extends into the wellness concept when companies screen for risk factors in addition to illness. Increasingly, corporate medical departments seek a balance between illness detection and risk factor identification in their screening programs. By incorporating the latest research on the medical efficacy of conducting each test on particular populations at given time intervals, employers try to determine what tests will have the most significant health impact and be cost-effective. Tests that are commonly performed at the worksite to detect high-risk populations include hypertension screening, breast cancer detection (often offered in the form of breast self-exam courses), glaucoma screening, sickle-cell anemia testing, blood tests, colon cancer screenings (frequently in the form of a self-administered test for blood in the stool), and height and weight measures for recognition of obesity. Most of these tests are low cost. Frequently, outside organizations such as the American Heart Association and the American Cancer Society, as well as insurance carriers, conduct these programs free of charge at the worksite as a community contribution or as a service to their clients.

The potential for risk reduction is great, as the programs of IBM and Pioneer Hi-Bred illustrate. Since 1968, IBM has had a multiphasic screening program that provides all 35-year-old employees with a battery of physical tests as well as a questionnaire that focuses on medical history and identifiable risk factors. Employees are eligible to repeat the exam every five years or whenever the IBM medical department suggests the tests are necessary. By 1980, approximately 90,000 employees had been screened (Beck 1980). The overall findings are striking. Of those screened, 41 percent had a previously unknown medical condition, another 33 percent had known conditions, and 26 percent were healthy based on the test results (Beck 1980). A breakdown of unknown vs. previously known is shown below:

Condition	Unknown	Previously known
Diabetes	112	1,588
Elevated sugar	10,061	1,776
Hypertension	3,494	8,368
Heart disease	3,075	3,762
Abnormal ECG	7,706	2,736
Blood chemistry	16,754	2,016
Uric acid	7,571	1,257
Cancer	89	938

Pioneer Hi-Bred in Des Moines, Iowa, is an example of a smaller company, with 2,500 employees, that implemented a health screening and incentive program in 1979, called Health Guard. All employees and their spouses are offered annual health screens, which include vital signs (pulse, temperature, and blood pressure), height, weight, and a urinalysis. A complete blood chemistry is done during their first screen. The screens are repeated annually for persons over age forty and for those with identified problems. Others receive these tests every five years. Results are confidential and are mailed to each employee or spouse along with a comprehensive explanation. The cost per person screened averages $48. Participation rates are 97 percent for employees and 70 percent for spouses.

The company reports several indicators of success in the four years that Health Guard has been operational. In 1979, serious abnormalities were identified for 6 percent of those screened, compared with less than 1 percent in 1982. In addition, during the first year the screens were conducted, the most prevalent conditions identified were, in order of frequency: hypertension, diabetes, cholesterol level and triglyceride level. Four years later, they were cholesterol level, tryglyceride level, hypertension, and diabetes. Pioneer also reports that many diabetics identified in the first screen are now being treated through diet and exercise modifications.

The disparity in the screening results between the IBM (41 percent unknown medical conditions) and Pioneer Hi-Bred (6 percent with severe abnormalities) reflects the varying levels of results that can be achieved through different screening programs. IBM's screening is vastly more inclusive and thus has a much greater opportunity to detect abnormalities. The two companies also defined abnormalities differently.

Control of Disease and Biological Risk

The workplace, with its regular schedules and the economic incentives to help people avoid leaving work to go to the doctor, is an ideal location for treatment or control of diseases that require continual monitoring over a long period of time where the monitoring can be performed safely outside a medical care setting. For example, Baltimore Gas & Electric's medical department screens for hypertension, educates hypertensive employees, follows up every three months to assure compliance with the treatment, and, if necessary, provides the medication. Two areas discussed below are hypertension control and employee assistance programs (EAP), for which the evidence of effectiveness is fairly strong.

Hypertension

The relationship between hypertension and mortality is well documented by the Framingham study. This epidemiological study of 6,507 individuals was designed to determine the relationship between a variety of presumed risk factors—including hypertension, high levels of cholesterol in the blood, obesity, lack of exercise, and smoking—and two major killers: diabetes and cardiovascular diseases. Named for the Massachusetts town in which the study has been conducted, the Framingham project is still collecting data after more than 30 years. One of the findings is that some 56 percent of those who died from cardiovascular disease were found to have a blood pressure of 160/95 or more, compared with 37 percent whose blood pressure was under 140/90 (Dawber 1980).

A recent study has produced results that are highly supportive of hypertension worksite programs. The University of Michigan's Institute for Labor and Industrial Relations, the Ford Motor Company, and the National Heart, Lung, and Blood Institute collaborated on a project to determine the relative effectiveness of four methods of hypertension referral and treatment programs (Erfurt and Foote 1983). Site one served as a control. The program consisted of hypertension

TABLE 6.1   Hypertension prevalence and control rates among Ford employees, University of Michigan project

	Site 1	Site 2	Site 3	Site 4
Employee population	2,561	4,619	4,316	3,502
Number screened	2,121	3,453	3,314	2,308
(% work force)	(83%)	(75%)	(77%)	(66%)
Prevalence of hypertension	16%	19%	17%	13%
Control rates: (blood pressure below 160/95)	(N=211)	(N=555)	(N=493)	(N=86)
Baseline	33%	36%	19%	24%
Final visit	47%	87%	90%	98%

Source: National Heart, Lung, and Blood Institute, *National Heart, Lung, and Blood Institute Demonstration Projects in Workplace High Blood Pressure Control* (draft paper prepared in May 1983).

screening and referral to the employee's doctor, if appropriate. Except for a courtesy letter to the physician, no follow-up was conducted until the end of the two-year trial period. Employees at site two were provided minimal follow-up, consisting of referral to the employee's physician with an accompanying letter to the physician and semiannual follow-up sessions. Employees at site three were provided full follow-up. The main difference between sites two and three was the intensity of follow-up. While employees at site two were contacted only on a semiannual basis, at site three follow-up visits were scheduled as needed according to the severity of hypertension. Employees at site four were offered complete hypertension treatment by the plant physician. Those not electing to accept on-site treatment were followed according to the site three protocol. The annual per-person cost of each program was $26 at site two, $35 at site three, and $96 at site four. The results of the two-year study indicated that site four provided the most successful treatment modality, as shown in table 6.1.

A correlation between the control of hypertension and absenteeism was also found. One year prior to screening, matched hypertensives were absent more than normotensives at all four sites (30, 28, 12, and 29 percent more for sites one through four, respectively). Hypertensive employees reduced their absence rate over the two-year period following screening in all three experimental sites. Active participants in sites two and four approximated that of normotensives by the second year. In contrast, absenteeism among hypertensive employees increased at the control site.

Employee Assistance Programs (EAPs)

Frequently an outgrowth of alcoholism programs, EAPs focus on emotional problems of employees that, if left unattended, can be precursors of more significant—and potentially more costly—psychiatric and physical health disorders. According to an unpublished 1982 Washington Business Group on Health survey, more than 75 percent of this group's membership, which includes predominantly Fortune 500 size employers, now offer some form of EAP. Some use in-house staff exclusively, others contract out for services, while still others do both. EAPs often result in referrals to private practitioners for ongoing treatment. Although many insurance plans discriminate against mental health services, particularly outpatient treatment, the basic insurance plan is still the payment mechanism for treatment that exceeds the limitations of the EAP. Standard Oil of California provides full coverage for mental health treatment, but only when it is recommended by the EAP staff.

The principal purpose of most programs now is to assist employees with personal problems (mental, legal, family, job-related, etc.) or illnesses (substance abuse, emotional illness) that can affect job performance. Employees may enter the program through self-referral or at the request of a supervisor who believes that job performance has declined. Frequently, the alternative to seeking help through the EAP, particularly where a substance abuse problem exists, is disciplinary action or dismissal. Many EAPs have expanded their focus on treatment or crisis intervention to include programs that help individuals effectively manage their time, stress, career, and family relationships to help prevent crises from occurring.

Employers have discovered that EAPs reduce accidents, absenteeism, and medical utilization, and also improve productivity. Further discussion of these benefits is included under Evidence of Effectiveness.

Detection of High-Risk Lifestyle

Many high-risk behaviors are the targets of public service messages provided by voluntary agencies, the government, and health organizations. Employers also provide information through newsletters, posters, audiovisuals, and pay stuffers. Health fairs have become popular community events combining the resources of many local groups to educate the public about health and risk factors. National leadership in the development of these fairs has been assumed by the nonprofit National Health Screening Council for Volunteer Organizations, Inc. (NHSCVO). This organization is the catalyst for media, corporate, volunteer, and public sector financial and in-kind services. In 1983, it involved more than 120 volunteers providing health screens across the country. The health fair has four components: health education, screening tests, referrals, and follow-up. Specialty programs are now offered to the elderly, minorities, students, the disabled, and local companies as part of a wellness strategy. Some employers, such as the Campbell Soup Company, have held health fairs for their own population to increase awareness of the dangers of high-risk behaviors and to assist with biological risk and disease detection.

In addition, statistical analyses have been performed of health risks that make it possible to determine an individual's relative risks (such as smoking, exercise, seat belt usage, weight, height, blood pressure, and reaction to stress) and provide him or her with an analysis aimed at assisting in behavior modification (Dunton and Fielding 1981). Many forms of these appraisals exist. They range from a one-page self-scoring form providing a synopsis of comparative risks, to very elaborate questionnaires yielding computer-generated responses such as risk age compared to actual age, projected life expectancy based on risks, and likelihood of illnesses that the high-risk individual may contract within five years.

Reduction of High-Risk Behavior

Employers use a variety of approaches to assist employees in reducing high-risk behaviors, including information dissemination, formal educational programs, behavior modification efforts, and financial incentives.

Information dissemination

Employers have adopted a variety of information dissemination techniques. Many companies (e.g., Kimberly-Clark, Xerox, Boeing) provide nutritional information in cafeterias listing calories and cholesterol content of food. Some companies (Ford, DuPont, Boeing) offer a special "heart healthy" menu. Citibank offers seminars for employees on the appropriate warm-up techniques for exercise, how to buy running shoes, and how to develop an exercise regimen. Ford posts maps of two of its corporate offices with mileage measurements for employees who wish to walk indoors during breaks. Armco developed an off-the-job safety program when it discovered that off-the-job accidents caused 427,457 days lost between 1966 and 1977, which was the equivalent of closing a 500-person plant for three years. The program consists of calendars that identify a safety topic for every month, flyers that are sent to employees' homes with safety tips, and meetings devoted to the safety tip of the month.

Education

Another approach is to conduct educational programs designed to alter personal behavior. Topics include nutrition, safety, maternal and child health, back care, driver safety, rape prevention, and alcohol and drug abuse. The distinction between information dissemination and education is that educational programs attempt to assist people over time by using more elaborate educational methods, such as repetition, reinforcement, personal contact, and the tailoring of information to appropriate learning levels. Companies such as Ford Motor Company, AT&T, and Metropolitan Life Insurance Company employ health educators. Other companies, such as IBM and Rolm, contract with community resources.

In addition, many employers have found self-help programs to be the most feasible method of providing employees education on behavior change. They are usually cheaper than classes, can be conducted at home where family members can participate, and can be offered at all work locations. Instruction methods range from workbooks to audiovisual or computer-taught courses.

One of the most extensive such programs is the Xerox Health Management Program, which entails written communication, incentives, and peer support. The employee is given a self-starter kit, which includes instructions on how to conduct a step-by-step fitness evaluation, begin a personal exercise program, cease smoking, and manage weight; there is also a bimonthly health management newsletter and posters are placed in work areas. Computerized health risk appraisals are provided. Employees are encouraged to participate and are assisted by worksite-trained volunteer facilitators. In April 1983, a buddy-system incentive program was initiated. Pairs of participants enter into a contract with each other stating that, by the end of the year, they will not smoke, be within ten pounds of ideal weight, and exercise at least three times per week. Employees who meet the contract terms receive a T-shirt. If the pair is still participating in the contract system after a certain number of months, they also each receive a wallet, and their names are placed in a drawing for items such as home computers and AM/FM stereo systems.

Behavior modification

Noneducational mechanisms of changing behavior are offered by some employers. These include hypnosis, mostly for smoking cessation and weight control (Massachusetts Mutual Life Insurance) and biofeedback to control reaction to stress through body monitoring (Equitable Life Assurance Society). Aversion therapy is sometimes used to help individuals stop smoking. The smoker, with guidance from a professional, smokes cigarettes continuously until it becomes unpleasant if not nauseating.

Financial incentives

An unpublished study of worksite-based behavior change incentives has identified 25 programs in 19 companies operating on or before July 1982 (Shepard and Pearlman 1982). Included were 15 smoking cessation, 5 weight loss, and 4 exercise and fitness programs, plus a stress management program. Some were offered in conjunction with behavior change assistance, while others were independent.

Analysis and Computer Systems offers monthly bonuses to those who quit smoking. The bonuses amount to $50 for the first 6 months after cessation and $300 for months 7 through 18. Six employees have participated in the program, all of whom successfully stopped. In 1967, City Federal Savings and Loan Association began paying all nonsmoking employees $20 per month extra. All nonsmokers qualified, regardless of whether they had ever smoked. Coors Industries provides a $45 rebate in $15 installments on a $60 smoking cessation program fee to those who quit for 12 months, $15 reimbursement for a slimness course, and up to $100 if weight loss goals are met during a nine-month period. Intermatic, Inc. matches up to $100 of smokers' self-placed bets on whether or not they will stop smoking. Successful quitters are also eligible for a trip to Las Vegas. In addition, four dollars per pound is paid for employees who meet their weight loss targets, and one dollar per pound is paid for those who do not meet their target but lose at least 15 pounds.

Hospital Corporation of America pays employees to engage in aerobic activities. Twenty-four cents is paid for each aerobic unit. Examples of units are one mile of walking or running, a quarter mile of swimming, four miles of biking, a quarter hour of aerobic dancing, and a half hour of racquetball. From June 1982 through June 1983, the company paid a total of $15,000 to the 300 corporate office employees who participated in the program. Twelve hundred were eligible to participate.

Pioneer Hi-Bred offers overweight employees and spouses five dollars per pound lost until the desired weight is reached. If the desired weight is maintained for one year, the participant has a choice of gifts valued at roughly $75. Of all overweight employees, 60 percent participated in the program, and 90 percent of the participants have lost at least some weight. The company also will pay an employee or spouse $150 to quit smoking for one year. A $75 gift is offered to the successful ex-smoker if abstinence is maintained for an additional year. An estimated 37 percent of the workforce smoked at the beginning of the program; 14 percent of these quit for two years as a result of it.

Blue Cross of Oregon offers an insurance plan that integrates a medical expense account (see chapter 2 on plan design) with a wellness program. In order to receive the unused portion of the account, the employee must participate in specified wellness activities and be absent from work one day less than the average of days missed by all employees.

Several companies offer incentives for seat belt usage. Teletype Corporation in Little Rock, Arkansas, randomly checks for seat belt usage as employees enter or leave the parking lot and awards wearers with coupons for McDonald's. General Motors has given away four cars through a seat belt incentive program. Employees sign a pledge that they will wear seat belts. When a certain percent of employees is found to be wearing seat belts as determined by a random check, a drawing for a new car is held for all who have signed pledge cards.

Many companies—e.g., Holiday Inn, Sentry Insurance, and Control Data Corporation—offer material incentives, such as T-shirts, books, gym shorts, and wristwatches, for achieving a desired health outcome.

Corporate Culture that Facilitates Healthy Behavior

Experts in the field of worksite wellness recognize the importance of a supportive environment. Corporate attitudes, management styles, methods of communication, and the physical environment all influence behavior. This section discusses three components of a cultural strategy: the physical environment, corporate leadership, and management style.

Physical environment

The work setting can be altered in many ways to facilitate healthy behavior, including making available facilities that promote physical fitness. In some people's perception, the presence of these facilities is synonymous with wellness programs. However, they are not essential for a successful wellness program, and evidence is lacking regarding whether or not they stimulate behavioral change, although they clearly are a convenience for employees.

There are many ways in which the workplace can be made conducive to good health. Nutritious, low calorie or low cholesterol foods can be made available in cafeterias and vending machines, and menus can include nutritional information. There can be showers to encourage exercise, bike racks to encourage bicycle commuting, and quiet rooms for meditation and other forms of stress management. Attractive decor and noise control can enhance well-being, as can smoking restrictions that protect nonsmokers from exposure to cigarette smoke and reinforce the desirability of not smoking.

Some companies, such as Kimberly-Clark in Neenah, Wisconsin, offer a full range of exercise options at the worksite. The facility in Neenah houses a swimming pool, a running track, saunas, a whirlpool, areas for exercise classes, and weight training. It is part of a comprehensive program consisting of four components: medical screening with exercise testing, health education, aerobic exercise and cardiac rehabilitation, and an employee assistance program.

One of the most extensive physical facilities is that of Coors Industries in Golden, Colorado. A few years ago, the company purchased and renovated a Safeway supermarket, which is now a wellness center. Activities at the wellness center include an extensive physical fitness program in which about one-third of employees participate; a stress management program, which includes classroom sessions and one-on-one counseling; a weight reduction program; a smoking cessation program; an extensive alcohol education program; and nutrition counseling. Many of these activities are open to family members. Vending machines have nutritious meals, with calories and cholesterol content marked. (Free beer is available, but it is limited to light beer.)

Leadership

Corporate leaders can contribute to the acceptance of a culture that promotes positive health lifestyles by personal example and by incorporating wellness principles in policies, corporate programs, and management styles. While many corporate leaders are responsible for wellness cultures, there are a few who have been one step ahead of the crowd or willing to make an exceptional commitment.

Darwin Smith, chairman of Kimberly-Clark Corporation, was personally responsible for the recruitment of the medical director,

Robert Dedmon, M.D., who pioneered the company's wellness program in Neenah, Wisconsin. The national attention received by Kimberly-Clark has led numerous companies to follow its example. James Burke, Chairman of Johnson and Johnson, declared that he wanted to have the healthiest workforce in the United States and, as a result, supported the development of the Live for Life program and encouraged J & J's commitment to sound research on the program's effects. The commitment of Thomas Frist, M.D., President of Hospital Corporation of America, to aerobic exercise led to the development of the company's aerobic financial incentive program and the building of the corporate gym. While only a fourth of the employees participate in this program, it is estimated that many more participate in other forms of wellness activities as the result of the example set by their leader. Dr. Frist is a marathon runner and is frequently seen running to and from work.

Management style

For years, there has been controversy over which management styles generate the greatest productivity. As information increases on the relationship between stress and health, there appears to be some logic to the belief that the style of the work environment will affect health. Management style, health, and productivity are all interrelated. One component of a management style that appears to transcend the attempt to maximize productivity and foster healthy lifestyles is the degree to which employees can contribute to their jobs and to the corporation, and the amount of control they have over their environment. Examples of employee control include active participation in the design and implementation of wellness programs, quality circles and other opportunities to provide input to the design or production of a product, and employee committees that focus on improving the environment so that healthy lifestyles will be facilitated.

Dennis Colacino, the director of fitness programs at PepsiCo, describes the integration of wellness into company culture in the following statement:

> Health is a reflection of our time and environment. At PepsiCo, we try to reach a philosophy that in fact reflects the time and environment. You are familiar with "Run America Run," "Catch that Pepsi Spirit," and "We've Got Your Taste For Life"—That's the emphasis of our program. Wellness is a posture in our corporation and part of our environment. It's not a fringe benefit.

PROVIDERS OF WORKSITE WELLNESS PROGRAMS

Starting in the mid-1970s, a host of organizations have targeted the workplace as a market for health promotion products. This section summarizes the efforts of some of the groups that offer worksite programs, specifically hospitals, voluntary organizations, the insurance industry, other private firms, the YMCA, and worksite wellness organizations. It also summarizes supportive efforts of foundations and coalitions.

Hospitals

The changing nature of illness, public attitudes about medical care, and competition within the medical care system have stimulated hospitals to expand their services to include wellness programs. A 1981 AHA survey showed that 53 percent of hospitals engage in some form of community health education, 59 percent provide a health education program for their own employees, and 13 percent offer services for a fee to industry (Jones 1981). The programs in the last category were wellness (9.3 percent of total), employee assistance (5.8 percent), and occupational health programs (7.2 percent). The major reasons expressed for initiating these programs were, in order, to improve community relations, to improve hospital relations with local business, and to develop a long-term revenue source.

Services designed for employers include many forms of testing services (e.g., pre-employment physicals, occupational hazard screens, fitness testing, and hypertension screening); courses that can be offered at the hospital or the worksite (e.g., stress management, exercise and physical fitness, smoking cessation, special diet programs, healthy back and proper lifting techniques, and nutrition); programs for high-risk populations such as working mothers, older workers, diabetics, and workers with sickle-cell anemia; rehabilitation; employee assistance programs; and on-the-job emergency medicine, such as cardiopulmonary resuscitation (CPR), Heimlich maneuver, crisis intervention, and how to stock a first aid station.

A 1982 AHA survey offers examples of hospital-based wellness activities that are oriented to the worksite (Bader et al. 1982). Overlook Hospital in Summit, New Jersey, conducts employee assistance programs for some 18,000 workers in 14 companies. The program was developed with government support from the National Institute on Alcohol Abuse and Alcoholism and was first tested on the hospital's employees. Union Hospital in Lynn, Massachusetts, has had 75 corporate and organizational clients. The most popular programs have been stress management and alcoholism. The Skokie Valley (Illinois) Community Hospital Good Health Program includes lifestyle assessments (computerized health risk assessment, physical screening, and a behavioral assessment) and health promotion workshops keyed to the results of the lifestyle assessments. Workshop topics include aerobic fitness, nutrition, weight control, stress management, smoking cessation, and cancer prevention. During periodic follow-up and evaluation, quantitative progress and impact measures compare the individual's health risks from one year to the next.

Franklin County Public Hospital in Greenfield, Massachusetts, provides occupational health and employee assistance services to 35 small employers. Lifestyle programs are planned for the near future. Pacific Medical Center in San Francisco offers a broad array of services, including CPR, worksite emergency planning, nutrition counseling, and compliance with the Occupational Health and Safety Administration (OSHA). These are provided both at the hospital and at local worksites.

Voluntary Organizations

Many voluntary agencies that formerly offered programs in the community now have taken their public education campaign and services to the worksite. Several factors have stimulated this change: many worksite programs have a track record of successfully detecting and following illness; the worksite presents a captive audience; and employers and employees contribute to many of the agencies by assisting in fund-raising drives.

For example, the American Lung Association provides smoking cessation assistance at the worksite through three mechanisms: courses taught by volunteers or staff members, training programs for worksite volunteers on how to conduct programs, and the distribution of the association's "Freedom From Smoking" self-help kit.

The American Cancer Society (ACS) offers a series of one-hour lectures on all forms of cancer. The series can be presented either by ACS staff members or by nurses or nonprofessional employee volunteers trained by ACS. The society also offers a smoking cessation course, which can be taught by volunteers or trained facilitators. A marketing package has been developed for volunteers to use when talking with employers about worksite cancer prevention and early screening programs. IBM and the Washington Business Group on Health have assisted in the development of these materials. A kit for corporate medical directors on how to design an internal cancer prevention and screening program has also been developed. Finally, ACS hosted the 1981 conference, "Smoking OR Health." A model smoking policy emerged from the worksite segment of the conference and is being distributed to employers.

The American Heart Association offers community programs that are available at the worksite, including hypertension screening, CPR, and nutrition courses. The association plans to increase its emphasis on worksite programs. The American Red Cross offers a selection of courses that can be conducted at the worksite, including hypertension control, CPR, nutrition, weight control, stress management, and accident prevention. The Red Cross has also developed "Guidelines for Health Promotion Programs in the Red Cross Workplace," which was distributed to all Red Cross sites in early 1983. The March of Dimes produced a program on birth defect prevention for working mothers. It is a self-contained kit with a manual and audiovisuals that can be used by a worksite trainer.

For each of these organizations, the programs are conducted through local affiliates and volunteers. The national association provides materials, training, and support. Programs are not offered uniformly across the nation, since resources and priorities of local affiliates vary.

The Insurance Industry

The insurance industry entered the worksite wellness movement with motivations that were similar to those of the hospital industry, i.e., to improve relations with employers as part of marketing strategy. Social responsibility has motivated some to participate; others have accepted wellness as part of their cost-management services. Many insurance companies also have programs for their own employees.

Individual insurance company endeavors include a campaign in business publications promoting worksite wellness sponsored by the Metropolitan Life Foundation; conferences on worksite wellness (Blue Cross/Blue Shield of North Carolina); consulting services for client companies (Metropolitan Life Insurance and several Blue Cross/Blue Shield plans); and printed materials and/or films to assist with program design and implementation (John Hancock, Prudential).

In addition to company programs, the two associations that represent the insurance industry have contributed to the worksite wellness movement. The Health Education Committee of the Health Insurance Association of America (HIAA) has helped foster individual company efforts by producing a booklet on the economic benefits of worksite wellness programs and by launching a smoking cessation initiative. This initiative entails the development of a model plan to reduce smoking, which will be implemented by the HIAA member carriers. These carriers will then assist client companies that want to implement the program. The HIAA, in cooperation with the American Council of Life Insurers, is also conducting an educational program for chief executive officers on the benefits of wellness programs. The program includes an audiovisual presentation highlighting corporate chairmen discussing the benefits of their programs.

The Blue Cross and Blue Shield Association provides member plans with assistance in developing worksite wellness programs for their own employees and subscribing companies. The association surveyed plan activity in 1982 and found that almost all of the plans are involved in some form of worksite wellness.

Other Private Firms

Like hospitals, insurance companies, and voluntary agencies, a variety of private firms have targeted employers as a market for wellness products. Products include comprehensive wellness programs that can be delivered nationally on-site (Control Data's STAYWELL Program); physical testing with courses and wellness activities in a resort setting (the Houstonian and the Sun Valley Institute); audiovisual presentations (Spectrum Films and McGraw-Hill); workbook programs (Bull Publishing); employee assistance programs (Human Affairs, Inc.); and courses and seminars on a large selection of topics sold by numerous individuals and businesses.

The Young Men's Christian Association (YMCA)

The YMCAs offer wellness programs to employers at many locations. The National YMCA Association also developed a working relationship with IBM to assist all of the company's facilities nationally to implement its Plan for Life program. Many local YMCAs have developed relationships with employers ranging from offering discounts for group purchases to coordinating a comprehensive wellness program that includes the use of other local resources. Many YMCAs have full-time staff devoted to worksite programs.

Worksite Wellness Organizations

Few national business organizations have made the promotion of worksite wellness a priority. One exception is the Washington

Business Group on Health, which, starting in the mid-1970s, has promoted the concept as an integral part of a corporate health strategy. Also, the Association for Fitness in Business promotes the expansion and improvement of worksite wellness through its 2,000 members.

In addition, several local organizations were formed in the early 80's for the specific purpose of promoting worksite wellness programs. One example is the Wellness Council of the Midlands, an organization of companies in Omaha, Nebraska that are combining resources to help other companies start and improve local programs. They produce a monthly newsletter, conduct seminars, and provide technical assistance. They have also produced and are airing a televised public service announcement. Another example is the San Diego Wellness at the Workplace project, conducted jointly by the California Governor's Council on Wellness and Physical Fitness and the San Diego Chapters of the American Heart Association and the Association for Fitness and Business. The project is designed to enhance the quality of worksite wellness programs by coordinating local resources.

Foundations

Some foundations have funded worksite wellness program development or evaluation. The W. K. Kellogg Foundation is funding the evaluation of the effectiveness of the wellness programs of Blue Cross of Indiana and Blue Cross and Blue Shield of Michigan. The foundation is also funding two community-based wellness programs that target the worksite for program implementation in Seattle, Washington and Williamsport, Pennsylvania.

Coalitions

More than two-thirds of the coalitions rank health education among their top five priorities. This is true regardless of the coalition's composition or stage of formation. Health education efforts include communication programs to assist employees in using their medical benefits prudently as well as in improving their health. Health education has not fully evolved yet, because most coalitions have as the top priority either developing a utilization data base or activist programs like health planning. However, wellness has been the subject of seminars and conferences for several coalitions, such as the New York Business Group on Health. As another example, the Lehigh Valley Business Group on Health has developed a four-component strategy to assist members in the development of wellness programs: (1) a conference for local wellness organizations to help them determine the services to offer business, (2) a seminar for business leaders on the rationale for implementing wellness programs, (3) a series of seminars on specific methods for implementing wellness programs, and (4) an ongoing resource center that distributes up-to-date information and houses a lending library.

EVIDENCE OF EFFECTIVENESS

The growth of worksite wellness programs, despite the dearth of scientifically valid evaluation, indicates that many employers believe in the concept's intrinsic value. Those who have initiated programs appear to be satisfied with the logic that healthier workers will be more productive workers. However, the increase in providers and programs has increased the press to discover which approaches will yield the greatest results. This information would assist an employer who wishes to make a commitment to wellness yet has concerns about the best way of spending limited resources. These limited resources are, however, one reason why more scientifically valid information does not exist. Most companies would rather devote funds to programs than to expensive evaluations.

There are several other factors that inhibit the evaluation of worksite wellness. Most worksite wellness programs that have been operational for more than a few years did not identify specific goals initially or adopt an evaluation strategy. Also, a company may have a multiplicity of goals, and employee morale, which is very difficult to quantify, may be as important as reduced medical, disability, on-the-job accident, turnover, or absenteeism costs. Although many programs can relate outcomes to change in knowledge, behavior, attitudes, or physical measurements, few evaluations to date can relate these changes to actual cost savings. Many of the measures that would logically be included in a cost-benefit evaluation of a wellness program are unavailable in most companies. For example, few companies track medical utilization for specific individuals. Many do not have comprehensive statistics on sick leave and, instead, only collect long-term absence data (five to ten consecutive workdays). Also, quantifiable measures of productivity are difficult to obtain. However, as corporate medical and personnel data systems improve, so does the ability to evaluate wellness programs.

Another difficulty is posed by the problem of developing valid control groups, since most companies will not deny programs to a control population for the purpose of evaluation. It is also a fact that carefully designed evaluation is expensive. Most corporate leaders who have made a commitment to wellness programs are satisfied that their investment is worthwhile and do not wish to expend the additional resources to find out exactly what the program has accomplished.

Two companies, Johnson & Johnson and Control Data Corporation, are making financial commitments to conduct scientifically valid evaluations that will help all companies understand the merits of wellness programs and determine which components produce the desired outcomes. These are discussed below, followed by a summary of some other studies.

Johnson & Johnson—Live for Life

Objectives of the Johnson & Johnson program include improvements in nutrition, weight control, stress management, fitness, smoking cessation, and health knowledge. Also, the proper utilization of such medical interventions as high blood pressure control and the employee assistance program is strongly encouraged. Employees are provided with a health risk screen and have the opportunity to participate in health enhancement programs at the worksite. Also, employee task forces are responsible for creating a work environment that supports positive health practices.

An essential element of the program is the annual health screen, which is available to all employees. The screen includes biometric variables (blood lipids, blood pressure, body fat, weight, and estimated maximum oxygen uptake), behavioral variables (smoking, alcohol use, physical activity, nutrition practices, coronary behavior pattern), and attitudinal measures (general well-being, ability to handle job stress, personal relations, organizational commitment, and job involvement).

Control groups were established for the evaluation. Some 2,100 employees at four Johnson & Johnson facilities with the Live for Life program were compared with 2,000 employees at locations without the program. The evaluation protocol compares the baseline screening results with the findings from two subsequent years. The first report was issued in late 1981 and is the source of the figures below. Results of the second year's comparison will be released in October 1984.

Significant findings of behaviorial changes include a 43 percent increase in aerobic calories burned measured in kilograms per week in the Live for Life population (the treatment sites) compared with a 6 percent increase in the control group, a 15 percent decrease in smoking at the treatment sites compared to a 4 percent decrease at the control sites, and a 1 percent decrease in the percentage of the population that is above ideal weight compared to a 6 percent increase in the control group. There was also a 32 percent reduction in the percentage of the population with elevated blood pressure compared with a 9 percent decrease at the control site, despite the absence of a program designed specifically for hypertension control.

The evaluation also measured changes in self-reported sick days and attitudes, as shown below:

	Treatment N=727	Control N=680
Self-reported sick days	−9%	14%
Satisfaction with working conditions	3	−7
Satisfaction with personal relations at work	1	−3
Ability to handle job strain	0	−2
Job involvement	2	0
Commitment to the organization	0	−2
Job self-esteem	0	−2
Satisfaction with growth opportunities	−1	−3

A preliminary study of the impact of the Live for Life program on medical utilization is also underway.

Control Data STAYWELL

STAYWELL was initiated in 1979 and is currently available to 22,000 Control Data employees and their spouses as a free employee benefit. It is also marketed to other companies as a commercial venture. Participation among Control Data employees ranges between 65 and 95 percent at the various site locations. The program includes a confidential health risk profile with a workshop to interpret the results, a health screen, one-hour overview courses on lifestyle and health, and comprehensive sessions given over periods of several weeks dealing with smoking cessation, stress management, weight control, nutrition, and fitness. Control Data also has employee participation groups that attempt to alter the work environment to promote healthy lifestyles, as does Johnson & Johnson.

Data for the evaluation are collected primarily through a survey administered to a 10 percent sample of all domestic Control Data employees (approximately 5,000 people). Employees at STAYWELL locations are compared to those at locations without the program. Respondents in the STAYWELL group are also subdivided based on whether they are nonparticipants, health risk profile participants only, participants in other activities but not in the extensive lifestyle classes, or participants in the lifestyle change course.

Control Data reports several positive effects. For example, smokers enrolled in the smoking cessation course smoked an average of 1.6 packs per day at the start of the course. Twelve months after the course, 30.3 percent were not smoking, 43.5 percent were smoking less than one pack per day, and 24.2 percent smoked one or more packs per day.

The evaluation also determined that people with poor health habits are 86 percent more likely to miss work and 100 percent more likely to limit the amount of work they do. They are also more likely to take prescription drugs. Finally, the Control Data evaluation confirmed the relation between health habits and health care benefit payments. For example, current smokers and those who quit less than five years earlier generated 25 percent more benefit payments and twice the number of hospital days as those who either never smoked or quit within the previous five years. Also, sedentary individuals experienced a claims cost that averaged $436.92 and .57 hospital days compared with $321.01 and .37 hospital days for the more active people.

Other Studies

There are also less scientifically valid studies that offer some indication of the benefits of worksite wellness programs. The most convincing of these relate to hypertension and smoking cessation. According to Jonathan Fielding, M.D., based on a review of available research:

> A voluntary on-site [hypertension] screening, referral, and follow-up program at the home office of Massachusetts Mutual Life Insurance Company led to an increase in the percentage under control from 36 percent to 82 percent after one year of operation.
>
> In a three-site industrial hypertension screening, detection, and follow-up program, 92 percent of 120 auto workers, 138 sanitation workers and 106 postal workers referred for high blood pressure saw their physician, and 93 percent of those seeing a physician had treatment initiated. Of those initiating treatment, about 84 percent showed progress towards control. In 28 Chicago-area hypertensive employees who attended a special high blood pressure control clinic near their work place, average diastolic blood pressure fell from 102.6 mm Hg at first screening and 98.8 mm Hg at second screening to 83.1 mm Hg at the end of the first year. (Fielding 1982)

Fielding also reports that smoking cessation programs at the worksite have achieved a 40–60 percent abstinence rate over a 6–12 month period, compared to 15–30 percent achieved through community programs.

For many employers, less rigorous evaluation of the positive impact that wellness programs can have on problems like absenteeism, turnover, and on-the-job accidents have been sufficient to gain their support. Some of the studies have estimated actual cost savings as a result of wellness strategies. However, we are not in a position to pass judgment on the validity of the results reported. Furthermore, companies may be more willing to report successes rather than failures.

New York Telephone, which has 80,000 employees, estimates an annual savings of $663,000 from its hypertension control program, $1,565,000 from its alcohol control program, $269,000 from its breast cancer screening program, $302,000 from its back treatment program, and $268,000 from its stress management program (Wood 1980). The Occidental Life Insurance Company and Northern Natural Gas Company report reduced absenteeism as a result of a fitness program. Canada Life Assurance found that program participants had a 1.5 percent turnover rate compared to a 15 percent rate for employees who did not participate. Forty-seven percent of fitness program participants reported that they were more alert, enjoyed their work more, and had better rapport with co-workers and supervisors since the program began. The National Aeronautics and Space Administration and the New York State Education Department have reported positive benefits in employee attitude, general sense of well-being, and reduction in absences as the result of fitness programs.

Kimberly-Clark reports a 70 percent reduction in on-the-job accidents among its EAP participants. The General Motors EAP has been used by 44,000 people in 130 locations. The company reports decreases among program participants of 40 percent in lost time, 60 percent in sickness and accident benefits, 50 percent in grievances, and 50 percent in on-the-job accidents (Berry 1981). Other cost savings from EAPs are shown in table 6.2.

ISSUES

Any field that is expanding at the rate of worksite wellness raises a number of complex and controversial issues that will take time to resolve. The most significant issue, evidence of effectiveness was addressed in the last section. This section discusses five other issues: confidentiality, illness liability, product line conflict of interest, competition and quality control, and the ethics of early detection.

TABLE 6.2   Cost savings reported for some employee assistance programs (EAPs)

Company	Number of employees	Number using EAP	Rehabilitation rate %	Annual cost savings
University of Missouri	7,000	1,002	80	$ 67,996*
Scovill Manufacturing	6,500	180	78	186,550
Illinois Bell Telephone	38,490	1,154	80	254,448†
(family)		100		
U.S. Postal Service	83,000	?	75	2,221,362
Kennecott Copper	7,000	1,200/yr.	NA	448,400‡
(with dependents)	28,000			
New York Transit	13,000	?	75	2,000,000
E.I. DuPont (with spouses)	16,000	176/yr.	70	419,200§
New York Telephone	80,000	300/yr.	85	1,565,000

Source: Charles A. Berry, *Good Health for Employers and Reduced Health Care Costs for Industry* (Washington, D.C.: Health Insurance Association of America, 1981), 28.

* Plus a 40% decrease in use of health benefits.

† 31,806 disability days were saved and off-duty accidents decreased 42.2% and on-duty accidents decreased 61.4%. There were also savings in health insurance utilization and job inefficiency.

‡ The total included absenteeism, sickness and accident disability, and health insurance use. Absenteeism decreased 53%, weekly indemnity costs (sick accident) 75%, and medical costs 55%. The rehabilitation rate was not calculated. A conservative calculation found a $5.78 return for each $1.00 invested in the program.

§ Alcohol program only.

Confidentiality

Both individual employees and union leaders have expressed concern about the confidentiality of health information. This issue encompasses information on medical claims, medical data collected during examinations, data from special services such as employee assistance programs and other forms of mental health treatment, and risk analysis collected through assessment tools. The concern is that this information may be misused in decisions about promotion, job assignment, or termination.

While it is generally agreed that employers should not have direct access to a given individual's health data, there are several benefits to both employees and employers from the company's receiving aggregate information. These include the ability to tailor interventions to meet actual need, to evaluate program effectiveness, and to spot unusual occurrences of illness or risks so that environmental causes can be detected. There are also instances in which information on individuals can be valuable. For example, preplacement physical examinations are conducted to determine whether someone is capable of handling a specific job, raising the issue of what constitutes being capable. One issue is whether companies should be allowed to screen employees for stress tolerance when placing them in a stressful job.

There appears to be a fine line between protecting the individual and protecting the company. As risk detection becomes more advanced through such methods as genetic screening, this issue will become more controversial. Current mechanisms of protecting individual data include: sending the results of screenings and risk assessments to employees at home and to the physician of their choice if requested; contracting with outside organizations, which in turn provide the company with aggregate data only; and establishing policies stipulating that only program staff will have access to information on individuals.

Illness Liability

Another complex issue is the determination of responsibility for illness caused or exacerbated by potentially controllable behavior, such as smoking. There is considerable professional debate about the degree to which many risk factors are controllable, especially for those at greatest risk, e.g., the heavily addicted smoker. Further, when someone hurts himself at play, or even when drunk, there is no suggestion that the price of recovery should be any different from that for unavoidable illness or injury. There is no clear definition of what constitutes illness that is wholly lifestyle dependent. Another aspect of this issue is the division of responsibility between employer and employee when the former provides a less than safe work environment and the latter knowingly adds to the problem by, for example, smoking. Coke oven, asbestos, and cotton dust exposure cases are often complicated by this dilemma.

Product Line Conflicts of Interest

Producers of products that are known health risks are forced to trade off the enhancement of their employees' health against the promotion of their product. The tobacco industry illustrates this point. The surgeon general has singled out smoking as the most preventable cause of death in the United States. However, most cigarette producers encourage their own employees to smoke by giving them free cigarettes, by not having nonsmoking areas, and by not offering smoking cessation assistance.

A classic example of this problem was recently reported in the *Wall Street Journal* (March 31, 1983). Heublein Inc., a liquor and food company, had designated smoking and nonsmoking sections at meetings. After they were acquired by R. J. Reynolds Industries, the nation's largest cigarette maker, the practice was stopped. A spokesman for Heublein explained, "We are owned by a company that has a significant position in the tobacco industry. We don't encourage employees to smoke, but we don't discourage them either."

Competition and Quality Control

The wellness movement is being pulled in conflicting directions. From one side come pressures demanding quality standards, an educational background tied to licensure, relative effectiveness measures, and all the trappings of an organized service delivery profession. Graduate degree programs are opening; reimbursement is increasingly available for selected services of wellness providers; corporate staffs are growing; and the skills of yesterday's narrowly focused fitness experts are expanding to include many aspects of health, medicine, education, and communication.

At the same time, physicians are looking for new areas of practice as a result of increasing supply and are entering the wellness market. In some cases, they are attempting to control the market by requiring a physician's authorization before participation in a fitness program or by linking reimbursement for smoking and weight reduction programs to doctors' orders.

The competition among providers is requiring purchasers to become increasingly more sophisticated so that they can make rational selections. It also requires greater effort to evaluate alternative programs and approaches.

Ethics of Early Detection

Early detection programs based upon increasingly elaborate screening have gained considerable acceptance in industry. Along with the obvious advantages of discovering a potentially serious (and expensive) illness at a stage when prevention can be effective, these screenings pose some challenging ethical problems.

For example, screenings given without a one-on-one educational session can contribute to anxiety and confusion, or to a false confidence, depending on the reported results. False positives are so frequent in some of the tests that high costs can result from the need to retest. In addition, there is otherwise unnecessary utilization and the risks associated with false positives. Finally, their psychological impact is almost impossible to measure, but all one has to do is to consider being told that one may have cancer and then waiting a week to get the results of a retest.

Screening often demonstrates that selected physician services, psychological counseling, nutritional and other lifestyle changes, or new drug therapies would contribute to prevention. However, these are also often the very services and providers for which the company insurance plan provides no reimbursement. One solution is to offer an array of in-house preventive services to assure that appropriate follow-up is not hindered by economic constraints that would not apply to acute care services.

As described in the discussion above on confidentiality, there is fear by some employees and unions that the results of screenings will be used by management for hiring, firing, and job assignment decisions, rather than for the provision of preventive care. Also, screening can identify a health problem and establish that its cause is the worksite itself, and some firms are more willing to screen than they are to correct the problems that are discovered. Only a major commitment by management and labor can bring about the needed changes to the physical environment and or corporate culture that will result in the prevention of future illness.

CONCLUSION

In 1970, only a handful of U.S. employers had initiated any programs that emphasized health promotion and disease prevention. By 1980, it would be conservative to say that 50 percent of the larger companies had established one or more programs called wellness. Today, worksite wellness programs are expanding in prevalence, in comprehensiveness, and in sophistication. Increasingly, smaller employers, public sector employers, unions, nonprofit sector employers, and hospitals are offering wellness programs or facilitating access to community services. This phenomenon mirrors the growth in general public commitment to healthier lifestyles and concern for the escalation of medical care costs.

The expansion of worksite wellness programs has not been based on data that demonstrate the financial return of the program, although some evidence does suggest that this can be one outcome. Rather, the expansion has emanated from the cultural acceptance of the changing nature of illness, greater understanding of limitations of the medical system, and the awareness that health can be promoted through behavioral and environmental changes.

As programs become more sophisticated, they will bring more cultural changes into the workplace. Many aspects of the changing society, such as family structure, values, and available resources, are already being integrated into the work environment. This can be seen through the development of day care centers, extended leave programs, retirement programs, programs for older workers, programs for working parents, flex-time, and the greater development of part-time working arrangements. The work setting is becoming more humanistic in nature and is focusing more on self-responsibility. Self-responsibility is the backbone of the wellness programs but can only be achieved if the environment, particularly the work environment, facilitates the behaviors that will achieve optimal health.

REFERENCES

Bader, B.S. *Planning Hospital Health Promotion Services for Business and Industry.* Chicago: American Hospital Association, 1982.

Bauer, K.G. *Improving the Chances for Health: Lifestyle Change and Health Evolution.* San Francisco: The National Center for Health Education, 1980.

Beck, R.N. "IBM Health Care Strategy." Presentation made to Council on Wage and Price Stability, 16 April 1980.

Berry, C.A. *Good Health for Employers and Reduced Health Care Costs for Industry.* Washington, D.C.: Health Insurance Institute, 1981.

Cardiovascular Primer for the Workplace. Washington, D.C.: National Heart, Lung, and Blood Institute; Office of Prevention, Education and Control; Health Education Branch, 1981 (NIH Publ. No. 81–2210).

Cunningham, R.M. *Wellness at Work.* Chicago: Blue Cross Association, 1982.

Dawber, T.R. *The Framingham Study.* Cambridge, Mass.: Harvard University Press, A Commonwealth Fund Book, 1980.

Dunton, S., and J. Fielding. *Promoting Health.* Chicago: American Hospital Association, 1981.

Erfurt, J.C., and A. Foote. *Final Report: Hypertension Control in the Worksetting—The University of Michigan Ford Motor Company Demonstration Project.* DHHS Contract No. N01-HV-8-2913. Submitted to the Heart, Lung, and Blood Institute, 1982.

Fielding, J.E. "Effectiveness of Employee Health Improvement Programs." *Journal of Occupational Medicine* 24(November 1982):907–916.

Jones, L. *AHA Special Selected Topic Survey Data—Employee Health.* Chicago: American Hospital Association, 1981.

Kiefhaber, A., and W. Goldbeck. "Smoking: A Challenge to Worksite Health Management." In proceedings, *The National Conference on Smoking OR Health: Developing a Blueprint for Action.* New York: American Cancer Society, 1981.

Kristein, M. "How Much Can Business Expect to Earn from Smoking Cessation." Paper presented at workshop, Smoking and the Workplace. National Interagency Council on Smoking and Health, Chicago, 9 January 1980.

Naditch, M.P. "The STAYWELL Program." In *Behavioral Health: A Handbook of Health Enhancement and Disease Prevention*, by J. P. Matarezzo et al. New York: John Wiley & Sons. In press.

National Center for Health Statistics. *Health United States, 1983*. DHHS Publication No. PHS 84-1232. Washington, D.C.: U.S. Government Printing Office, 1983.

National Heart Lung and Blood Institute Demonstration Projects in Workplace High Blood Pressure Control. Draft paper prepared May 1983. (For further information contact Judith H. LaRosa, NHLBI, Building 31, Room 4A18, Bethesda, MD 20205.)

Shepard, D.S., and L.A. Pearlman. *Incentives for Health Promotion at the Workplace: A Review of Programs and Their Results*. Boston: Center for the Analysis of Health Practices, Harvard School of Public Health, No. 677, 1982.

Weis, W.L. "Can You Afford to Hire Smokers?" *Personnel Administrator* 26(May 1981): 71-73, 75-78.

Wood, L. "Lifestyle Management Strategies at New York Telephone." Paper presented at the Leadership Strategies-Health Conference, Millwood, Va.: Project Hope, 1980.

7

In-House Corporate Medical Programs*

Diana Chapman Walsh
and Eileen J. Tell

PERSPECTIVES ON INDUSTRY'S DIRECT
DELIVERY OF HEALTH CARE

For many years a sharp line has been drawn that excludes any illness
or injury unrelated to work from the scope of occupational medicine.
The line was drawn by the American Medical Association, respected
by industrial physicians, and deferred to by corporate executives.
However, in practice, the distinction between occupational and nonoccupational illness has always been elusive, and it was only with respect to job-related industrial accidents that the distinction was ever
clear-cut. In an era of chronic degenerative disease, the traditional
lines separating occupational from nonoccupational diseases are becoming increasingly blurred.

Reflecting this blurring, a number of large corporations have
gradually expanded their capabilities for servicing employees' primary health care needs. These expanded in-house programs often
begin with the hiring of part-time specialists—for example, internists, dermatologists, orthopedists, or psychiatrists—and informing
employees that they are welcome to use the medical department for
advice about and treatment of minor problems. More serious or
chronic problems are still referred out, either to the employee's personal physician or to one recommended by the medical department.

*Portions of this chapter have been adapted from (Walsh 1984).

Relations with the private physicians of employees are handled gingerly and on a case-by-case basis, although the expansion of the inhouse service is frequently undertaken after the company becomes aware that many of its employees do not have a personal physician.

Opinion is divided as to the merits of expanding the mission of corporate medical departments to include personal health care. Advocates believe it makes sense both economically and medically (Sahin and Taylor 1979). They contend that the corporate medical department is capable of performing a variety of routine tests and procedures more efficiently and as effectively as anyone else. The convenience of the medical department reduces time away from work, and a high quality comprehensive health program is good for morale and for the department's credibility with employees. It also allows corporate physicians to practice their clinical skills, which in turn enables the corporation to recruit first-rate practitioners (Greer et al. 1977). Advocates of the approach consider it the surest way to upgrade the status of occupational medicine.

Critics challenge both the economic and the medical premises. They assert that companies that provide extensive primary care services may pay twice, since there is no way of knowing whether the employee's visit to the expanded medical department is an adjunct or an alternative to the use of outside medical services. Firms offering extensive primary care services have not been able to demonstrate a measurable impact on health care premiums, nor have they substantiated the claim that the convenience factor saves time away from work. Also, most large firms are too widely dispersed geographically for the approach to be practical in more than one or two highly concentrated locations and few, if any, moderately sized or small firms can justify the expense of an elaborate in-house medical service. The critics believe the corporation should allocate its finite health dollars to preventive occupational health programs that do not duplicate services available on the outside (Schilling 1981). Some see occupational medicine in the vanguard of a new national strategy of health promotion and disease prevention and worry that a focus on primary health care will cause companies to dilute their own efforts or undercut the existing community health infrastructure.

Between the advocates and the critics there is a middle ground, with corporate medical staff serving a brokering and watchdog function. They maintain collegial ties with an extensive outside network of health care providers. They examine some or all levels of employees on a periodic basis (e.g., once every two or three years) and refer out those with positive findings for follow-up care. Not doctrinaire in eschewing a primary care role, they willingly do needed testing or follow-up requested by employees or their outside physicians but leave the initiative with the employee and his or her personal physician. They help monitor quality by keeping a watchful eye on the claim forms that come through for short-term disability and try to provide a subtle but decisive second opinion when they think an ill or disabled employee may be getting poor medical advice.

It is on this middle ground that most large, well-established corporate medical programs stand. A certain amount of primary health care seems unavoidable. Even in England, where there is a strong ideological bias against company sponsorship of comprehensive medical services as inimical to the spirit and vitality of the National Health Service, a national commission has estimated that one-third of the time of industrial health practitioners is devoted to "casualty work and treatment . . . the sort of work undertaken by general practitioners in the NHS"—work the commission explicitly excluded from its definition of occupational medicine (Robens 1972).

If the corporate medical department has had a circumscribed role, so has the benefits staff. Until very recently it has been the rare company that has seen those two functions as anything but entirely separate. To the benefits specialist has fallen the task of designing the plan, negotiating premiums and administrative terms with the carrier, and administering the benefits program. The medical services themselves, particularly their utilization, have been perceived as beyond the legitimate control of the firm. Concerns about health care costs, therefore, focused initially on administrative arrangements—retention rates, cash flow, and interest on the reserves built up to pay claims. The advent of new forms of contracting, such as administrative services only, minimum premium plans, and self-administration of claims, were greeted with much excitement (Egdahl and Walsh 1979). However, decisions to adopt these new contracting forms did not entail medical judgments and thus were properly made without significant involvement of corporate medical departments.

The key change that is now underway relates to the willingness of the corporation to manage its benefits, including passing judgment on the appropriateness of utilization review systems, participating in processes to determine the appropriate supply levels for beds and services in the community, channeling patients to particular providers, and developing wellness programs. Benefits managers have also been increasingly concerned with the integration of planning for health benefits with other areas such as disability determination, the development of rehabilitation plans for individual employees, and sick leave management. These new roles for the benefits manager all share a common characteristic: implicitly or explicitly, they entail medical judgments, inevitably raising new questions about the role of the corporate medical department.

TABLE 7.1   Possible missions and strategies for corporate health

Mission	Related strategies
Containing workers' compensation and liability costs	Emergency treatment for occupational incidents Accident prevention Workplace monitoring for toxic substance levels Workplace monitoring for stressors Ergonomics Research into occupational disease (toxicology, epidemiology) Stewardship of product safety Control of environmental pollution and toxic waste disposal Preemployment and preplacement examinations Periodic examinations of exposed workers
Compliance with regulatory requirements	Toxicological testing of new substances Workplace monitoring of toxic substance levels Accident prevention Periodic examinations of exposed workers
Improving employee relations	Periodic examinations (nonoccupational conditions) Workplace monitoring for stressors Health promotion and fitness programs Counseling and employee assistance
Improving employee productivity	Any or all of above plus primary care
Containing health benefit costs	Administering/monitoring health benefits Periodic examinations (nonoccupational conditions) Health promotion/employee assistance Accident prevention/workplace monitoring Primary care Activities in outside health care system (alternative delivery systems, coalitions, utilization review)

Source: Reprinted with permission from Egdahl and Walsh's *Corporate Medical Departments: A Changing Agenda?*, Copyright 1983, Ballinger Publishing Company.

A taxonomy of major activities of corporate medical departments is presented in table 7.1 (Egdahl and Walsh 1983). The first two missions, "containing workers' compensation and liability costs" and "compliance with regulatory requirements," are within the purview of the department's traditional functions. The last three—"improving employee relations," "improving employee productivity," and "containing health benefit cost"—are largely new functions.

From the standpoint of medical care, the most interventionist activity of the corporate medical department is that of offering a range of ambulatory health services as a presumed alternative to care the employee would otherwise have purchased with benefit dollars on the open medical market. It is to this topic that the remainder of this chapter is devoted. The four case studies presented deal with the programs of the Gillette Company, which has an active program of primary care; Gates Rubber Company, which has established a direct delivery program for employees and dependents; Public Service Gas and Electric Company of Colorado, which has an HMO-like program called an Employees Mutual Aid Association; and New York Telephone Company, which has developed and begun to evaluate a health care management program.

It should be borne in mind that all of the programs described are relatively longstanding. They are initiatives only in the sense that they are unusual, rather than because they are new, and in the sense that they might be considered precursors of a possible trend as companies become more aggressively involved in the overall management of health care costs. On the other hand, it is still the prevailing view in occupational medicine that the direct delivery of primary health care services is a deflection from the discipline's central mission. The case studies here raise interesting issues concerning the future of corporate medical departments. It should also be noted that a number of unions—e.g., United Mine Workers, International Ladies' Garment Workers Union—have provided services through their own clinics. These are not discussed in this chapter.

THE GILLETTE COMPANY

The cardinal feature distinguishing Gillette from most other companies is its explicit commitment to providing a wide range of personal health services for acute and chronic illness, whether or not associated with conditions at work. In 1980 Gillette employed 33,900 people worldwide, operated 50 plants, and distributed its products in 200 countries. Just over 6,000 employees, or about 18 percent of the total workforce, are located in the Boston area, the site of its corporate headquarters.

For employees in Boston, Gillette supports three medical facilities. The largest is in South Boston. It was constructed in 1952, serves some 3,500 employees, and has five salaried physicians plus an additional seven who have hourly contracts. All 12 physicians are board-certified or board-eligible. Five are internists with specialties in the areas of hematology, gastroenterology, endocrinology, allergies, and diabetology. Two are surgeons, four are ophthalmologists, and one is a dermatologist. Gillette physicians, unlike most other corporate medical doctors, also maintain private fee-for-service office practices in the community. All are active members of the medical staff of University Hospital and have appointments on the faculty of Boston University Medical School.

The clinic is staffed around the clock, with nurse coverage for the two night shifts. There are seven registered nurses, three of whom are certified nurse practitioners. Physicians are on call at all times. If an employee on a night shift requires immediate medical attention, the Gillette nurse on duty sends him or her to the emergency room of the Boston University Hospital, where all of the Gillette physicians have staff privileges. The hospital nurses contact whichever of the Gillette physicians is on call at that time.

The two other facilities serve about 1,200 and about 1,600 employees. These facilities rely primarily on nurses to provide first-line primary care, with back-up from the medical staff at the South Boston clinic.

Because of their ties with University Hospital, Gillette physicians are usually able to function as attending physicians for hospitalized employees. (Over 95 percent of Boston-based Gillette employees who were hospitalized in 1979 went to University Hospital.) This continuity of care throughout an episode of illness, together with the ability to see families of employees, is central to Gillette's claim that its medical program delivers an unusually personalized form of medical care (Greer et al. 1977). In addition, Gillette physicians believe that group practice elements, such as shared medical charts and overlapping responsibilities, promote effective peer review within their own system.

Most Boston-based Gillette employees (the company says more than 85 percent), including the chief executive and the majority of senior managers, use these physicians as their regular source of care. Employees who use the clinic do not face cost-sharing, whereas they face deductibles and coinsurance under the company's Blue Cross/ Blue Shield plan if they use private doctors. Thus, the clinic doctors in effect become a preferred provider organization (PPO). Dependents are not eligible to use the Gillette clinics, but many use Gillette physicians as part of their private practice and are reimbursed under the company's Blue Cross and Blue Shield plan.

Gillette physicians are convinced that their program has saved money. Rough estimates were made of the proportion of visits to the corporate medical department that would have resulted in a visit to an outside provider. The study concluded that $1.9 million in medical costs were avoided in 1976, as contrasted with operating costs for the clinic of $700,000. On the other hand, Gillette insurance premiums are not significantly different from those of other employers in the area, although detailed analyses have not been performed. In particular, the impact on services that Gillette does not provide directly (e.g., hospitalization) has not been carefully examined. One advantage of Gillette's program is that the company has the potential for analyzing costs in greater depth and being able to bring about changes more readily than would be the case if they were not providing services directly.

THE GATES RUBBER COMPANY

The Gates Rubber Company in Denver operates a comprehensive in-house medical center for employees, dependents, and retirees. The Gates Medical and Dental Center is located in a freestanding facility within the company complex. The clinic building, which has over 30,000 square feet of space, was built in 1963.

The clinic staff includes 17 full-time and 60 part-time physicians; 7 full-time dentists; and 115 nurses, technicians, assistants, and auxillary personnel. The internal medicine department includes seven full-time physicians, and there are four full-time pediatricians. Part-time physicians represent the following sub-specialties: allergy, dermatology, obstetrics/gynecology, neurology, oncology/hematology, orthopedics, osteopathy, otolaryngology, pathology, psychiatry, radiology, surgery, and urology. Other on-site services include a 24-hour first aid department, a fully stocked pharmacy, and a privately run optical shop that rents space from the Gates Medical Center.

The medical facility serves primarily Gates employees, dependents, and retirees, who are estimated to number 13,500. This represents 80 percent of the total population served at the medical center. The other 20 percent of patients are seen under contracts with other companies in the area. The Gates Medical Center provides first-aid and emergency services, medical care related to workers' compensation, and pre-employment physicals for about 75 other companies (including Montgomery Ward, Safeway, King Soopers, and General Iron). Also, Gates physicians may see private patients at the Gates facility.

Membership in the Gates Mutual Benefit Club entitles employees and their families to use the Medical Center and receive inpatient services and other benefits (such as life insurance). Employees' dues to the Gates Mutual Benefit Club serve, in effect, as their contributions to the health insurance plan. The level of contribution is modest: $3.60 per week, regardless of family size. Employees may also purchase major medical coverage, which has a weekly premium contribution of $9 per family and also has deductibles and coinsurance. However, there is no cost-sharing if company doctors are used. An estimated 60 percent of dependents and over 90 percent of employees use company doctors.

There is no cost-sharing for hospital services as such and no cost-sharing for inpatient services provided by Gates physicians. Enrollees who use other than a Gates doctor at Mercy Hospital do not face cost-sharing, because the doctors there have all agreed not to bill patients over the amount that the company recognizes as reasonable. The company also has a contract with Mercy Hospital which provides that, in exchange for semimonthly payments, Gates receives roughly a 20 percent discount on inpatient charges. Gates has also negotiated smaller discounts (3 to 4 percent) at other area hospitals which their employees may use. The majority of inpatient days, however, occur at Mercy. Thus, as with Gillette, Gates has in effect created a PPO arrangement.

Gates prides itself on its ability to attract and maintain highly skilled and well-respected physicians from the Denver community. The company attributes its success to the following: payment on a fee-for-service basis as opposed to a salaried arrangement, reduced paperwork, flexible scheduling of hours, prompt payment, and accommodations for physicians to see their private patients at the Gates Medical Center. In addition to their fee-for-service payments, physicians are entitled to a bonus if medical costs are controlled. The Gates medical program, however, is expensive. In 1982, the average cost was $2,752 per employee.

Gates periodically introduces changes in its services or benefit design. Increasingly, the medical program is contracting with outside providers for certain services rather than providing them directly. For example, it has entered into contracts with Mercy Hospital for after-hours emergency care, nutrition services, and speech and physical therapy. The transition to outside contracts has been made gradually. When physicians providing services have left Gates, they have not been replaced. Gates is also considering contracting for laboratory work and radiology.

Another unusual feature is the availability of prescription drugs at no charge. The Gates-operated pharmacy fills over 500 prescriptions a day, making it the largest pharmacy in Denver. After-hours prescriptions can be filled at King Soopers, a local supermarket chain. Employee response to the free prescription program has been very positive.

How does the Gates Medical Center measure up in terms of its cost-containment potential? The program has not been formally evaluated. However, Gates managers believe they are providing a more comprehensive benefit package at a cost comparable to, or below, the norm for other area employers. They also believe that the program has had a positive impact on absenteeism and productivity. Because of the proximity of the Center, employees lose less work time when they make a medical/dental visit. A good relationship between the medical department and factory management is also believed to enhance attendance and productivity. Physicians on a weekly basis monitor workers who are on compensation, disability, or sick leave. These physicians are presumed to be more knowledgeable of the demands of the work environment than are physicians in the general community. Gates physicians also feel that costs are saved since employees are less likely to have prolonged or more complex illnesses because of periodic examinations, prompt treatment, and thorough aftercare.

The current program structure was initiated before World War II, when medical services were not readily available and accessible in the community. Would the Gates Corporation establish a full-scale Medical Center today if such a program were not already in place? Probably not, the company's managers say. The program is costly to establish and maintain; many services that should be profitable are operating in the red; and hospitalization costs continue to soar.

What does the future hold for the Gates Medical Center? The company has considered expanding the site and opening up a greater portion of business to the general public. This notion has been resisted, however, by managers who feel that it is not appropriate for the Gates Corporation to compete in the health care business. In contrast, services are gradually being contracted out, which suggests that Gates might become less involved in the direct delivery of health care. Some Gates managers state that they cannot become less involved in direct medical care delivery because they would meet with intense employee resistance if the company clinic were scaled down or disbanded; however, there is talk that some Gates employees are unhappy with the current structure and would prefer to go elsewhere. Furthermore, some providers in Denver report a growing patient load of Gates employees.

PUBLIC SERVICE COMPANY OF COLORADO

The Public Service Company (PSC) of Colorado, an electric and gas company, has 6,800 employees, of whom 4,800 are located in Denver. Dependents of employees are provided comprehensive coverage through Blue Cross and Blue Shield, along with the option of joining an HMO. However, employees, other than those who join an HMO, are offered Blue Cross coverage only. Instead of being covered by Blue Shield, physicians' services are provided mostly by physicians who are employed by the company or upon referral by them.

The program, referred to as the Employees Mutual Aid Association (MAA), was initiated in 1907. It is now a separate nonprofit corporation with 501(c)9 status. The association has 11 board members, who are elected by employees and who represent the major organizational divisions within the company. The board appoints the administrator and medical director, who report directly to them. In addition to the medical director, there are six salaried physicians, five nurses, a pharmacist, a laboratory technician, and five clerical and secretarial staff.

The physicians are employed roughly half-time by the association and are salaried (except for one semiretired physician, the previous medical director, who works less than half-time). They have separate fee-for-service practices in the community. All physician services to employees are provided either by them or on referral by them. Although formal statistics are not collected, roughly half of all physician services are estimated to be upon referral. When a referral doctor recommends hospitalization, the admitting doctor is always an MAA doctor and not the referral doctor, thus allowing MAA physicians to maintain control over hospitalization. Most inpatient care is provided at St. Luke's, a major Denver teaching hospital, where the MAA medical director is also head of the emergency room. As with an HMO, services that are not provided by an MAA doctor or upon appropriate referral are not reimbursed at all, except for emergency and out-of-area services.

Services by the medical department are free to the employee. The first $1,200 of referral services to physicians are fully reimbursed. The patient faces 25 percent coinsurance for expenses between $1,200 and $3,200 (yielding a maximum in out-of-pocket expenses of $500). Above $3,200, there is no cost-sharing. Claims for referral services are processed by MAA. The administrative functions, including claims processing, are performed by the administrator plus five clerical staff. Hospital claims are processed by Blue Cross.

In addition, there is a company pharmacy, which dispenses the more commonly prescribed drugs. Employees can either use the pharmacy or take the prescription to a community pharmacy.

Arrangements vary for employees outside of Denver. In some communities, the association has agreements with a panel of physicians who are paid fee-for-service and who perform the same function as company physicians. In remote areas, employees can use any doctor.

Limited data are available to evaluate the program. Data are not kept on referral patterns of company physicians or on the practice styles of the physicians to whom they refer, nor are data available on hospital utilization. However, the costs of the total program are known, including fully allocated overhead. The one important item that is not allocated to the program is the fringe benefit cost of the medical staff, which is borne directly by the company. The per enrollee costs are somewhat above HMO costs in the area and thus are below what they would have been had the company relied on standard insurance coverage instead of the program they have. In 1983, these costs, including the Blue Cross component, were estimated at $76 per employee per month, compared with $70 for CompreCare and $59.70 for Kaiser, the two HMOs available to employees.

Not surprisingly, the major complaint of employees relates to the lack of choice of physicians. However, company representatives point out that many dependents voluntarily see MAA physicians as part of their fee-for-service practice. Furthermore, employees do have the option of enrolling in the two HMOs mentioned above, but fewer than 4 percent have done so. One of these (CompreCare) is an individual practice association (IPA) HMO with broad provider participation throughout the Denver region and would tend to attract any disgruntled employees.

NEW YORK TELEPHONE COMPANY

To serve its 80,000 employees throughout the state, the medical department at New York Telephone (NYT) employs 234 professional, paraprofessional, and support personnel. Of these, 40 are nurses, and physicians number 39 full-time equivalents. The company's health costs are estimated to have exceeded $209 million in 1981 and continue to rise at a rate of about 15 to 20 percent a year. The $209 million includes the costs of disability absence ($32.4 million), incidental absence ($20.9 million), health insurance ($103.6 million), workers' compensation ($4.7 million), replacements for lost time ($20 million), dental insurance ($18.8 million), and the costs of running the medical department ($9.1 million in 1981).

NYT's in-house medical program is directed by Gilbeart H. Collings, Jr., M.D., who believes that a medical department, to justify its existence, must contribute to the management of all health-related costs. Thus, the program differs from the three described above in that the company not only delivers care but also has an active program of focusing on preventive measures and disease interventions that have the greatest health status yield. It seeks to deal most effectively with identified disease, and it also strives to reduce the amount of future disease and to enhance the wellness or coping abilities of the firm's employees. An integrated data system is being built to facilitate future assessments of the efficiency and effectiveness of alternative strategies to conserve and enhance employees' health.

Dealing effectively with identified disease implies that the company's physicians will find a way to oversee the personal health care of the company's employees. How to accomplish that is a problem with which Collings and his associates have been struggling for a decade and a half. As a consequence, they have gone further than most corporate physicians toward specifying and even redefining the influence occupational medicine can hope to have on the personal health care system (Collings 1977, 1982).

To deal more effectively with established disease, improvements in case management are considered essential for controlling excess costs. Both case management and primary care services are delivered at eight principal locations and a number of secondary facilities throughout New York State. These are expected to deliver high quality health services to improve employee health, resolve or minimize the adverse effects of ill health and incapacity on company operations, and support operating management in day-to-day resolution of health problems.

The commitment to tackle the broadly defined problem of health-related costs has led NYT physicians to develop a concept they refer to as health care management, or HCM. Collings says HCM "discards a 50-year tradition which had limited occupational medicine to concern with job-related matters and had excluded it from significant involvement in the personal health of employees." He grants, however, "that others are moving in the same direction, that it is a matter of degree." Collings adds the further caveat that, unlike firms in more hazardous industries, the telephone company can allocate a large proportion of its medical resource to general health maintenance as distinct from environmental health concerns. HCM is conceived of as having three levels.

Level One: Correcting Clinical Malfunctions

On the first level, NYT physicians intervene in situations where they find malfunctions in the present clinical system. These may involve mistakes on the part of the employee's personal physician (improper or no diagnosis, inadequate or harmful treatment, excessive costs). They may also involve abuse of the system, in the form of excessive absence or employee noncompliance. Finally, they may involve inappropriate or unnecessary costs for hospitalization, surgery or ambulatory care. In each instance, the company physicians provide not therapy but management of situations in which established disease is being handled inefficiently or ineffectively.

NYT estimates that about 60 percent of the company's employees visit the medical department for one reason or another during the course of a year. Some rely on company physicians to guide them in their use of other practitioners, whereas others do not; the proportion that does is not known. The company's physicians seek gradually to develop relationships with employees. They do not ask them to sign up for health care management, nor do they even use that term with employees.

Level Two: Targeted Preventive Interventions

Once an employee begins to look to the corporate physicians for help in "getting healthy when they're not and staying healthy when they are," a so-called lifetime health strategy is developed. It begins with an initial baseline evaluation and is upgraded as experience accumulates.

The preventive strategies are individualized, and this is viewed as the key not only to case-by-case success but also to macroefficiency. For example, offering Pap smears annually for all 40,000 NYT women employees would cost about a half million dollars and yield perhaps three cases of disability averted owing to early detection of cervical cancer at a cost per case averted of $250,000. Instead, Pap smears are offered only to 5,000 or so high-risk women (based on race, heredity, sexual practices, age and other factors), thereby reducing the cost of the testing program to about $75,000 a year, for the same yield, at $25,000 per case averted.

Level Three: Advancing the State of the Art

For the longer term, and not yet implemented, health care management is seen as a practical management tool as well as a possible mechanism to advance the state of the art in preventive medicine. In theory, it should provide the means for integrating all available information on an individual's health and health practices over a working lifetime and for entering those into a data base where they can be compared with statistical norms. The statistical insights are used to modify and improve the individual's lifetime health strategy. Meanwhile, over a period of years, those experiences with individuals are aggregated and a knowledge base built so that high-risk individuals can be identified and high-yield interventions developed and applied. Thus, the corporate medical data base is viewed as a rich resource for applied epidemiological studies (Robinson and Wood 1982).

Overall Impact

NYT physicians believe that HCM is economically justified. (Many of its components are part of the wellness activities of a large number of employers and are described at greater length in chapter 6.) Based on preliminary data and projections, savings in costs and lives have been estimated, as shown in table 7.2. Clearly, these estimates will be refined over time. For now they are among the most elaborate cost-effectiveness estimates that any corporate medical department has unveiled.

CONCLUSIONS AND ISSUES FOR THE FUTURE

A preliminary assessment of the potential for the expansion of corporate medical departments into innovative programs that will enhance a company's ability to monitor the quality and the costs of care raises many questions. Companies have little incentive to publicize their efforts in this realm and many reasons to be circumspect. Occupational health is a politically charged arena. Corporate medical departments that have been able to overcome the profession's history of strained relations and to win the trust of both the company's employees and community physicians are understandably reluctant to rock the boat by calling attention to cost containment as an overt goal. Also, practitioners of occupational medicine are just beginning to examine their role and that of medical departments in constraining rising health care costs.

Direct delivery can be viewed as one end of a continuum in that it offers the greatest potential, if not the reality, for controlling utilization. In between direct delivery and the traditional laissez-faire approach to the ongoing management (or nonmanagement) of health benefits are such activities as utilization review, the selection or oversight of providers that participate in PPOs, and the design and administration of worksite wellness programs.

Companies that have been innovative in the delivery of personal health services seem to have done so more out of a desire to improve services to employees than to save money. Indeed, it is disappointing that their cost impact, as well as the quality of services provided, have not been studied more systematically. Furthermore,

TABLE 7.2   New York Telephone Company summary of savings from fully implemented health care management

	Annual dollars saved	Annual lives saved
SPECIFIC PROGRAMS		
Primary Prevention		
Fitness training	$ 103,300	2
Smoking cessation:		
Cardiovascular effects	645,400	13
Pulmonary effects	1,388,600	2
Cholesterol reduction	240,500	5
Hypertension control	663,000	12
Healthy back program	302,400	
Stress management	267,900	
Hemocult screening	85,800	4
Breast cancer program	269,000	6
	3,965,900	44
Secondary Prevention		
Alcoholism rehabilitation	$1,565,700	
High-incidence disease	979,000	
Pregnancy disability	800,000	
	3,344,700	
GENERAL HCM SAVINGS		
Absence from unspecified causes	$3,450,000	
Overtime cost reduction	1,200,000	
Hospital cost reduction	880,000	
Medical treatments that would have been charged to major medical insurance	495,000	
	6,025,000	
	$13,335,600	
Less: Program costs	−5,494,000	
NET SAVINGS	$7,841,600	

Source: Internal document, 1980.

whether they do save money or not may relate less to how they are structured than how they are managed. Meanwhile, occupational medicine's growing interest in health risk appraisal, health promotion, and data systems to monitor workplace exposures and their effects is reducing barriers between occupational and nonoccupational health problems. It seems probable, therefore, that there is more innovation—or at least more innovative thinking—now taking place privately than is apparent.

REFERENCES

Collings, G.H. "Health—A Corporate Dilemma; Health Care Management—A Corporate Solution." In *Background Papers on Industry's Changing Role in Health Care Delivery*, edited by R.H. Egdahl. New York: Springer-Verlag, 1977.

————. "Managing the Health of the Employee." *Journal of Occupational Medicine* 24(January, 1982):15–17.

Egdahl, R.H., and D.C. Walsh, eds. *Containing Health Benefit Costs: The Self-Insurance Option*. New York: Springer-Verlag, 1979.

————. *The Corporate Medical Department: A Changing Agenda?* Boston: Ballinger, 1983.

Greer, W.E., W. Kantowitz, and P.S. White. "Comprehensive Care through Physicians Serving in Both Corporate and Private Practice." In *Background Papers on Industry's Changing Role in Health Care Delivery*, edited by R.H. Egdahl. New York: Springer-Verlag, 1977.

Robens, L. *Safety and Health at Work: Report of the Committee 1970–1972*. Report presented to Parliament by the Secretary of State for Employment. London: Her Majesty's Stationery Office, 1972.

Robinson, H., and L.W. Wood. "The New York Telephone Company Medical Information System. *Journal of Occupational Medicine* 24(October, 1982): 840–843.

Sahin, K.E., and A.K. Taylor. "Employee Acquisition of Health Care Facilities: A Possible Outcome of Escalating Premiums?" *Sloan Management Review* (Summer 1979):61–75.

Schilling, R.S.F., ed. *Occupational Health Practice*. London: Butterworths, 1981.

Walsh, D.C. "Is There a Doctor In-house?" *Harvard Business Review* (July 1984).

8

Efforts of Trustees of Nonprofit Hospitals

Peter D. Fox

INTRODUCTION

There is evidence that the role of trustees of nonprofit hospitals is changing. Trustees are increasingly concerned with cost containment, and are increasingly willing to take a broader community view that extends beyond the purview of the single institution.

State rate setting and reimbursement limits in Medicare and Medicaid have had an effect, as have employer interests in encouraging boards to be aware of cost issues. Also, there has been increased competition by HMOs, other hospitals, and physician groups that are entering markets traditionally served by the hospital, such as ambulatory surgery and high-technology diagnostic services. These changes in the external environment have prompted recognition of the need for strategic planning. Cost containment has become an objective.

Boards of trustees are reasserting their roles vis-à-vis administrations. Court decisions that more clearly make trustees responsible for hospital affairs have played a part in this, as has the growth in regional multihospital systems, which give trustees a vantage point that extends beyond the individual institution.

These trends are likely to accelerate as a result of the very significant changes in purchaser practices, including Medicare reimbursement changes; the growth in contracts with health maintenance organizations, preferred provider organizations, and other competitive delivery systems; and various private purchaser initiatives to control hospital costs such as more stringent utilization review.

An integral part of the changing roles of trustees is efforts of large corporations vis-à-vis employees who serve as trustees, reflecting the perspective that companies have a legitimate vested interest in the positions and actions of employees on hospital boards. Many corporate executives have commented that trustees all too often leave their business acumen outside the door of the hospital boardroom.

A few companies (e.g., Owens-Illinois) have a formal policy of encouraging employees to serve on hospital as well as coalition boards, and many companies have well over 100 employees on hospital boards throughout the country, regardless of whether the corporate headquarters has such a policy. As an integral part of their cost-management strategy, some companies also provide training for these trustees, either by convening conferences at the company or by sending employees to various training programs. The extent to which these programs address cost-containment issues varies, as does the attitude of companies. Some companies simply want employees to acquire a broad perspective of the hospital and its relation to the community and are less concerned with whether cost issues are specifically addressed. Others want to ensure that there is a focus on cost issues.

The remainder of this chapter describes a number of the training programs that are being, or have been, conducted and then presents examples of trustee action.

EXAMPLES OF TRUSTEE TRAINING PROGRAMS

The Midwest Business Group on Health (MBGH) provides a good example of educational effort directed at hospital trustees. It has promoted trustee education efforts throughout the Midwest. MBGH first became involved in trustee activities by encouraging the establishment of the Hospital Trustee Planning Group in Rockford, Illinois. This group, composed predominantly of business people and cosponsored by the MBGH and the chamber of commerce, several years ago developed a series of educational sessions for trustees. Initially, the sessions were full-day affairs, but they evolved into two-hour morning meetings, scheduled every six weeks. Topics covered include health care regulations, HMO development, medical technology, and medical ethics.

Another example is the Trustee Week program sponsored by the University of Washington under a Kellogg Foundation grant. Trustee Week consists of a week-long series of workshops for hospital trustees, administrators, and medical staff in which individuals select those workshops best suited to their experience, interests, and board responsibilities. The various workshops assume different knowledge levels of participants, and trustees are encouraged to return in subsequent years. The program has been offered annually in the northwest since 1980 and was conducted in southern California for the first time in 1982.

The workshops are conducted in succession during the week so that an individual can attend more than one. The orientation workshop is a one-and-one-half day session at the beginning of the week covering the basic functions and duties of governing board members. It is geared to newly appointed board members. The intermediate workshop is geared to experienced board members or those who have had the orientation session. This two-day session in the middle of the week covers financial management, quality assurance, the hospital's mission, and policy making. There are also specialized workshops that provide two days of in-depth study in a particular area of concern to board members. They are offered at the end of the week. Workshop topics have included financial management, quality assurance, and the governing board's role in long-range planning. A substantial number of board members have returned in subsequent years and some hospitals have, over time, sent several trustees.

The University of Minnesota Trustee Education Program offers two-day seminars. Some of the sessions have been conducted for specific companies, e.g., TRW, Alcoa. The number of attendees at each session has ranged between 12 and 400. The first day of the seminar is devoted to developing a conceptual framework in which trustees can consider issues affecting their hospitals. Topics include the responsibilities and functions of trusteeship, social policy, finance, organizing forces, manpower, and the practice of trusteeship. The second day addresses specific management problems. Cost containment is not a major focus, and in a recent survey of attendees, only 10 percent identified cost control as a significant concern.

In 1981 and 1982, Deere and Company conducted two-day sessions for its executives who were members of hospital or other health-related boards. Each session has had about 30-35 attendees. The first day focused on financial management, strategic planning, marketing, multihospital relationships, and hospital productivity. Lecturers emphasized the similarities and differences in the application of these techniques between the management issues of a hospital and those of the company. For example, long-range planning was discussed in both contexts. The second day included a discussion of Deere's activities to contain costs as well as keynote speeches by invited guests who discussed trends and influences in the health care system, the fiduciary responsibility of a trustee, and other topics. In an effort to increase the visibility of health benefits issues to senior executives, all officers and directors of the company were invited to participate in several of the second-day sessions.

EXAMPLES OF SPECIFIC TRUSTEE ACTIONS

Innovative trustee actions can occur within a single institution or entail collaboration across institutions. Some communities have vehicles, such as coalitions, trustee councils, and hospital associations, that convene trustees from multiple institutions.

Some hospitals have taken measures, in advance of tight reimbursement controls, to constrain their costs. For example, the trustees of one hospital in Florida requested of their executives that the budget for 1983 not exceed the budget for the prior year, meaning that the full effect of inflation had to be absorbed.

Another hospital, in Illinois, which had expanded considerably during the 1970's, began to address cost issues in 1979. There were no specific external pressures, although the trustees could foresee the possibility of tougher Medicare controls, the enactment of a state prospective payment system, and the increasing prevalence of HMOs. For the last couple of years, they have kept the budget increases to 8 percent annually, compared to prior experience of 16 percent. In order to achieve the 8 percent target, departmental budgets were established in advance. They report no difficulty in achieving the savings.

Commonly, university hospitals report directly to the regents of the university. However, many have boards of trustees that are advisory to the regents. In 1982 the University of Minnesota president and regents charged the university hospital's advisory board, which was chaired by a retired insurance company executive, with recommending economies. One such economy was the scaling down in the size of a planned building program from approximately $190 million to $135 million.

In 1981, the Ohio State University Hospital implemented a new hospital governance structure, which included representation of the Columbus business community. One of the first actions taken was to freeze the hospital's charge structure and insist on certain economies. These decisions were heavily influenced by the impact, locally, of the hospital's costs on health insurance premiums.

An example of joint activity of trustees is that of two hospital councils, in Minneapolis and St. Paul, Minnesota, which were formed in late 1977 and early 1978 and which evolved out of pressures from the local HSA and the Citizens League, a voluntary good government group in the Twin Cities. They are known, respectively, as the West Metro Hospital Trustee Council and the East Metro Hospital Trustee Council. Each has a full-time staff. The West Metro Council established three task forces to address bed reduction, financial incentives, and miscellaneous issues such as health promotion and the consolidation of specialty services. The bed reduction task force recommended that hospitals voluntarily decrease the bed capacity by 1,100. Bed reduction in the community has occurred, although the actual contribution of the trustee organizations is difficult to measure because of other events and pressures in the community. In 1982, the council issued a report recommending that hospitals pursue such strategies as the release of hospital diagnostic-specific price and quality data, the adoption of common billing formats, merger and closures of services and facilities, and the promotion of alternatives to inpatient care. The East Metro Council has supported these actions, and both councils have active educational programs. In July 1982 all of the Twin City hospitals with more than 100 beds released price information for 25 diagnoses, and physicians in the area have started to post prices.

Hospital trustees in Rockford, Illinois, through their hospital trustee planning group, formed the Rockford Council for Affordable Health Care. Its membership includes most of the planning group as well as the chief executive officers of the three Rockford hospitals and representation from the medical society and insurers. The council has addressed such issues as the sharing of laboratory services among hospitals, new capital acquisitions, improving utilization review, and redesigning benefits. We have been told that, although the council does not have direct authority over hospital activities, it has been influential.

Other joint trustee activities have entailed developing new reimbursement systems. In 1978, the Rochester Area Hospitals' Corporation (RAHC) was formed in Rochester, N.Y., reflecting the culmination of a long history of trustee cooperation and concern with cost containment. The RAHC board is composed of two trustees from each of the eight hospitals in Rochester and from the University of Rochester Schools of Medicine and Dentistry. It assumed a lead role in working with administrators and area physicians to develop the Hospital Experimental Payments (HEP) program, which prospectively sets budgets for hospital expenditures in the area and then allocates these budgets to individual hospitals. Waivers were obtained from the New York State reimbursement program and from the Health Care Financing Administration in order to substitute HEP for usual Medicare and Medicaid reimbursement approaches and for the state rate-setting process.

In Maryland, trustees rather than administrators comprise the board of the Maryland Hospital Association. In 1971 they were largely responsible for the initiation of the Health Services Cost Review Commission, which runs one of the first rate-setting programs in the country.

Recently, the new Massachusetts rate-setting program, while originated largely by the business community and insurers, had widespread support among hospital trustees, many of whom are also business people.

CONCLUSION

A central issue is what should be the primary responsibility of trustees. Is it to promote the interests, narrowly defined, of the individual hospital or, instead, the interests of the community? If the latter, what role should cost-containment objectives play? Cost containment has not been a natural objective of hospitals. However, if trustees are to represent community interests, improving efficiency and eliminating unnecessary or duplicative services should compete with hospital expansion as priorities. Some trustees are accepting the fact that their interests may not always be congruent with those of administrators.

Also at issue is whether corporations that try to influence the behavior of employees who serve on boards create potential conflicts of interests. Do these employees owe their allegiance as trustees to the corporation or to the hospital? Corporate involvement can be viewed as a continuum ranging from no involvement whatsoever to the influencing of specific hospital decisions. Intermediate degrees of involvement may consist of encouraging employees to serve on boards and encouraging trustees to attend training programs. Most of these training programs do not emphasize cost containment but are likely to do so in the future as a result of recent Medicare changes and other pressures. Corporations can also try to ensure that trustees understand the need for institutional efficiency and are aware of the costs created by excess capacity.

The parallels and differences between hospital trustees and those of private, for-profit corporations are interesting. The responsibility of the corporation's board is to promote the profitability of the corporation, subject to the usual obligations of not violating legal or ethical standards. Social good is presumed to be maximized through self-interest guided by Adam Smith's "invisible hand." Interlocking directorates between a company and its supplier (in this case, the hospital) are often scrutinized by agencies responsible for antitrust enforcement. The hospital, however, is typically seen in a different light. The objectives and responsibilities of trustees are not always clear, and it is generally accepted that an insurance-based financing system does not promote an appropriate level of price competition or incentives for efficiency. Thus, it may be perfectly appropriate for corporations to seek a measure of influence through hospital boards over their suppliers of health care.

It is also worth noting that employees of corporations who serve as trustees do not always share a commonality of interest, any more than they always agree on matters that are unrelated to hospital affairs. For example, hospital boards often take positions on whether the state should have a rate-setting program. Corporations are often divided on this issue, especially in states where Blue Cross pays considerably less than full charges. Rate setting often results in the payment differential between Blue Cross and the commercial companies being narrowed, which in turn can result in premium increases for groups covered by Blue Cross and decreases for those covered by commercial insurance. As a result, corporations covered by Blue Cross are more likely to oppose rate setting, while those insured by a commercial carrier are more likely to favor it.

Finally, influencing trustees, either directly on specific issues or indirectly through educational efforts, has not been a high priority of most coalitions, nor has the formation of multihospital trustee councils, which provide a vehicle for purchaser communication with trustees as a group. In the future, it is likely that purchasers, through coalitions, will increasingly seek to influence trustee actions. One natural arena for coalition and trustee collaboration is in bringing about reductions in excess beds and services.

9

Towards a Purchaser Cost-Containment Strategy

Peter D. Fox

INTRODUCTION

Most companies are not in the health business. They are in the automobile, computer, communications, truck, chemical, steel, or other business. According to General Electric executive Linde E. Saline, "We know more about what goes into the cost of the 75-cent box of screws we use on the factory floor than we know about what goes into the cost of health care" (quoted in Louis S. Richman, "Health benefits come under the knife," *Fortune*, May 2, 1983). However, times are changing. Currently, considerable mutual education is occurring. More relevant data is becoming available for program management purposes, as is more information on the impact of potential changes. A small but increasing number of employers have taken action, and their successes are being watched and emulated.

This book has discussed the major private sector health care initiatives, concentrating heavily on those that purchasers can undertake. Some purchasers have limited their efforts to a single initiative —commonly, plan design. However, purchasers who will be the most successful in managing their health benefits will evolve a comprehensive strategy rather than adopting a single approach.

The elements of this strategy can be classified into three categories. The first such elements are those that the purchaser takes alone, such as plan design and the development of a worksite wellness program. In addition, a carefully structured employee communications program is vital in fostering an understanding of cost issues and in creating a corporate culture that reduces employee resistance to cost containment efforts. Such a program can also promote healthy behavior, help employees understand their benefits, and provide information on how they can be informed shoppers for medical care, e.g., by knowing how to elicit price information, select providers, and obtain a second medical opinion for surgery.

The second set of strategic elements entails actions that virtually require joint action among purchasers, such as through coalitions. These actions include community health education, the promotion of legislative changes, and participation in local facilities planning and other efforts to reduce the fixed costs associated with unnecessary capacity.

Finally, there is an intermediate set of measures that purchasers can adopt in isolation but that are more effective if undertaken jointly. These include developing comparative data bases on providers, conducting utilization review, negotiating with providers, and promoting HMOs and PPOs. Providers will, in most instances, be more responsive to demands for data on practice pattern changes when these demands issue from many purchasers rather than from an individual one; it is usually easier politically for purchasers to take certain actions jointly rather than singly.

The potential for combining utilization review, plan redesign, and enrollee communications programs illustrates the interactions among different initiatives. Many employers are changing their plans with the objective of reducing hospital use. Changes include increased cost-sharing for short stays, the introduction of second surgical opinion programs, coverage of ambulatory surgery, and penalties for weekend admissions. However, these changes will have greater effect if they are accompanied by utilization review to encourage providers to adopt efficient practice styles and by employee and provider education.

ILLUSTRATIVE STRATEGIES

The strategies that two companies—Deere and Co. and Owens-Illinois—have adopted serve to illustrate comprehensive strategies, each geared to the company's unique circumstances. Deere, a farm equipment manufacturer with 50,000 employees, switched to a self-funded and self-administered benefit program in 1971. However, as discussed in chapter 2, neither self-insuring nor performing one's own claims processing, in isolation, leads to cost containment, although savings may result from better controls on financial reserves and the exemption from premium taxes. Recognizing this, in 1977 Deere created its health care department, which now has a ten-person professional staff knowledgeable in health care management issues. The department, working with other company executives, evolved a strategy that includes

— Data Management. Deere has developed specifications for data that hospitals must report on claims forms before payment is made. Data elements include diagnosis and procedural codes, provider identifier, patient data, dates of treatment, and charges. These data allow Deere to profile the price and utilization experience of providers.

— Utilization Review. This corporation was one of the first in the United States to contract with peer review organizations for utilization review. Contracts have been signed with the Iowa Foundation for Medical Care and the Mid-State Foundation for Medical Care in Illinois. Utilization reductions of more than 30 percent have been realized, most of which is attributable to UR. Deere also heads the Business Advisory Council of the Iowa Foundation for Medical Care.

— Alternative Delivery Systems. The company has developed two IPA-type HMOs in Waterloo, Iowa, and the Quad Cities area. It has also assisted in the development of two other HMOs: the new SHARE Health Plan in Des Moines and a physician-sponsored IPA–HMO in Dubuque.

— Participation in Joint Purchaser Activities. Deere representatives sit on local coalitions around the state of Iowa, the board of the Iowa Health Policy Corporation, and the board of the Washington Business Group on Health. They also chair the Midwest Business Group on Health and co-chair the Governor's Commission on Health Care Costs in Iowa.

One impressive indication of the success of the Deere program is that the rate of increase in health benefit payments has been held below that of the consumer price index in each of the years since the formation of the company's health care department; previously, the rate of increase was about twice the CPI growth. Importantly, their achievements were realized primarily by affecting utilization patterns rather than through benefit reductions or major plan design changes. Critical to their success has been the support of top management, including the willingness of the chief executive officer to articulate clearly to the local provider leadership the seriousness of the corporate commitment to restraining inflation in health care costs.

Owens-Illinois is headquartered in Toledo, Ohio. It has roughly 100 manufacturing facilities in the United States and total U.S. employment of some 35,000. Operating under the explicit assumption that no single effort on behalf of a company or a community would adequately address the cost of health care, it has formally adopted a nine-point strategy.

— Top management support has been clearly articulated at the level of the chief executive officer and the board of directors. One element of this support was the establishment in June 1982 of the Health Care Policy and Programs Department.

— Employees are encouraged to serve on boards and committees of hospitals, Blue Cross and Blue Shield plans, HMOs, planning agencies, and other organizations involved in health care delivery.

— There is active participation in coalitions.

— Support for health planning includes corporate contributions to planning agencies. A particular focus of the company's emphasis on health planning is to limit capital spending that is likely to generate excess capacity.

— The company promotes enrollment in HMOs in order to create a more cost-sensitive market.

— It monitors legislation at federal, state, and local levels with regard to such programs as Medicare, Medicaid, and workers compensation. The company is also active in the Washington Business Group on Health, The Business Roundtable's Health Initiatives Task Force, and state chamber of commerce health care committees.

— It promotes employee understanding of benefits, including the desirability of considering alternatives to hospitalization, such as home health services and ambulatory surgery. The company also undertakes an employee education program to promote good health habits.

— Another aspect of the strategy is benefit package redesign. Effective January 1983, cost sharing was increased modestly, and several new incentives were introduced, including financial penalties for inpatient surgery that can be performed on an ambulatory basis, an incentive second opinion program for 13 elective procedures, and penalties for use of emergency rooms for nonemergency situations.

— In communities where the company has a high concentration of employees, utilization review is conducted. For example, the company not only contracts with PSROs but also employs its own medical staff to monitor utilization review activities.

SOME CONSIDERATIONS IN FORMULATING A COST-MANAGEMENT STRATEGY

Typical elements of a comprehensive cost-management strategy include: (1) the need to manage benefits, (2) changes in roles of the benefits and medical departments, (3) a clear identification of the problems to be addressed, (4) a recognition of the importance of data, (5) a recognition of the need to reduce fixed cost through capacity reduction in many communities, and (6) the need for top management support.

A recurring theme in this book has been the need of large purchasers not only to be prudent purchasers of benefits but also to manage their benefits. For example, home health benefits are most likely to serve as a substitute for hospitalization if the employer oversees the discharge planning process. Utilization review will be most successful if the company does not just contract out for review but also carefully monitors the review process, demands certain outcomes, and is prepared to conduct the review directly or shift to another review organization. Purchasers seeking to generate savings by contracting with a preferred provider organization (PPO) if results are not achieved need to understand PPO operations sufficiently to be assured of effective utilization review and that plan design incentives favor efficient over inefficient providers. As a final example, employers in areas of high employment concentration may find that they need to involve themselves in issues of capital spending and excess capacity.

One implication of the evolution of the cost-containment management function in the health care field is the assumption—of recent origin—that health benefits costs are at least partially controllable. An issue for multilocational corporations relates to internal incentive structure in the allocation of costs to profit centers. Some companies view health benefits as an overall corporate expense beyond the control of the individual plant or division manager and thus allocate health benefit costs based on a formula, e.g., as a percent of payroll. Doing so fails to incorporate incentives below the corporate level for management to constrain health care costs. In contrast, other companies charge individual units with their actual claims experience, which does provide incentives.

The implementation of a cost-containment strategy will entail expanded roles for the health benefits manager, who, traditionally, has not been expected to address such matters as data systems; health planning; the integration of health benefits with wellness, disability, sick leave, and other programs; decisions on alternative delivery systems; complex government relations issues; and so forth. Many of the elements of the strategies described represent new functions. In addition, greater integration of the employee health benefits staff and the corporate medical department is inevitable. Managing health benefits entails understanding and interacting with the medical delivery process. This, in turn, requires interpreting data about medical care and negotiating with providers. Furthermore, as employers become more enmeshed in utilization review and in channeling patients to particular providers, judgments about quality of care and the appropriateness of utilization will be necessary. These activities require medical expertise, albeit not of the type that all corporate medical departments currently have.

A clear identification of the problem and targets of opportunity are also important. The nature of the cost-containment problem varies among companies and communities and is heavily dependent on local provider structures and practice patterns. Not all communities have the same problems to the same degree. They vary, for example, in whether they rank high or low on admission rates, and in length of stay and use of ancillaries. They vary in terms of the local provider structure, the existence of viable local peer review organizations, the presence of HMOs, and the attitudes of other employers and state and local governments. Individual companies also differ with regard to such factors as the extent and nature of unionization, traditional practices on cost-sharing and premium sharing, the nature of employee relations, and the geographic concentration of employment. These differences, which are both analytic and political/sociological in nature, need to be reflected in implementation strategies.

Facilitating the process of problem identification are the enhancements, of recent origin, in both data availability and the ability of purchasers to specify the data that they really need and can use. Stimulated by the 1982 and 1983 legislative changes in Medicare, data have become readily available on the relative efficiency of individual hospitals, and many purchasers are contracting with firms that specialize in analyzing hospital utilization data. These data vastly enhance the ability of purchasers to assess the efficiency of hospitals by making possible valid comparisons of relative costs per case or admission, adjusted for diagnosis and other patient-related characteristics. However, they are not suitable for evaluating physician practice patterns outside of the hospital setting or whether the admission was in fact necessary. Data on physician practice patterns are harder to obtain, but they can be assembled, even if they are imperfect. This availability of data permits purchasers to make informed decisions—or, at least, educated guesses—regarding provider efficiency.

These data have many applications. They are of value for plan design, design of wellness programs, and health planning. In addition, an improved data base on physician charges can allow physician fee screens to be potentially set at a lower level than at present but with assurance that they are not below amounts charged by a significant proportion of physicians. Finally, improved data become the basis for distinguishing between efficient and inefficient providers. Employees can then be advised as to which providers are efficient, although this information is most likely to influence the behavior of employees only if they face cost-sharing. The findings are also useful in determining which providers merit inclusion in PPOs and in negotiating with providers over price or utilization. Measures can be adopted (such as reimbursement policies) to channel patients to efficient providers and away from inefficient ones.

A comprehensive cost-containment strategy must also address the problems of excess capacity. As one purchaser reduces the use of expensive facilities—whether through utilization review, promotion of ambulatory surgery or home health benefits, increased patient cost-sharing, or other means—large fixed costs can remain. In competitive markets, excess capacity leads to price competition, which, in turn, drives firms or suppliers out of the market. The extent to which classical economic theory is relevant to health care markets has been questioned. Nonetheless, the problems of excess capacity in the health sector can be addressed in a variety of ways, including marketplace competition, reimbursement limitations imposed by both public and private payers, public utility or health planning models, public pressure or suasion, and payer influence on hospitals boards. Which approach, or combination of approaches, is likely to be most successful, and the appropriate role of private purchasers, is a matter of some debate.

Finally, important to any company's strategy is the support of senior management and the communication of that support to employees, benefits managers, community leaders, and providers. Top management also needs to be aware that an effective cost-management strategy will likely entail greater coordination among various corporate departments than has historically been the case, e.g., benefits staff, the medical department, the finance staff, and the occupational health and safety staff. On the other hand, it is not essential that chief executive officers personally devote a lot of time to health benefits, although they do need to make sure that mechanisms are in place to address problems as they arise.

CONCLUSION

There is much that remains unknown regarding the impact of many of the initiatives, either because they are too new (e.g., PPOs), because no one has bothered to study them (incentives for ambulatory surgery), or because they are inherently difficult to study (e.g., coalitions). Furthermore, research is complicated by the potential interactions among initiatives (e.g., whether or not the promotion of care outside the hospital is combined with efforts to reduce inpatient capacity). In addition, the impact of many of the initiatives depends less on their structural characteristics than on how they are managed. Utilization review and PPOs are good examples of initiatives whose success depends less on their structural characteristics than on the commitment of the key actors involved and on day-to-day, often mundane, management decisions and style.

Finally, large corporations account for a minority of private group purchasing power, although they are usually the trend-setters, both because they can afford the staff necessary to innovate and because smaller employers often emulate them in order to attract workers in competitive labor and product markets. Roughly one-half of all employees work in firms with fewer than 100 employees. Another important group is comprised of the union-management (Taft-Hartley) and multiemployer trust funds. (These two groups clearly overlap: many employees of small firms are covered through trust fund arrangements.) Government at all levels purchases health benefits for its employees and has the potential, as employer, for exercising its purchasing power. The joint exercise of purchasing power of all these groups has enormous unrealized potential.

Epilogue

Peter D. Fox, Willis B. Goldbeck, and Jacob J. Spies

INTRODUCTION

Most of the research for this book was conducted in 1983. A major reason for our writing it—and for the U.S. Department of Health and Human Services sponsoring the research—was the pace at which private purchasers were innovating. Indeed, employers and unions are taking measures that would barely have been conceivable a few years ago. Furthermore, their new willingness to manage health care costs is permanent and will not lessen in times of high employment or low inflation.

Needless to say, changes have continued to occur since our manuscript was prepared, although we have incorporated some additional data and examples throughout the editing process. This epilogue seeks to capture selected, but important, aspects of the changing environment as this book goes to press in the summer of 1984.

BENEFIT DESIGN

Some changes that were highly innovative two years ago are becoming increasingly commonplace. Incentive second opinion for surgery programs—i.e., programs with cost sharing penalties if second opinions are not obtained—are being widely adopted, and all employers are seeking to shift the locus of care to ambulatory settings where feasible. Most employers would like to neutralize the cost sharing structure to avoid incentives to use the hospital; some are more successful than others, depending on employee relations, union strength and attitudes, and relations with carriers, particularly Blue Cross plans that pay considerably less than full billed charges.

In chapter 2 we discussed a program with an innovative cost sharing structure that relates deductible levels to wages, introduced by two employers, Jones & Laughlin and Xerox. Although hardly a groundswell, other employers (e.g., Alcoa) are examining this structure, and at least one, Baxter Travenol, has recently adopted it. Under the Baxter Travenol plan, the deductible is 0.5 percent of wages. For most expenses above the deductible, the employee faces 10 percent coinsurance on ambulatory services and 20 percent coinsurance on inpatient services. This creates incentives to avoid using the hospital.

Companies that have adopted medical expense accounts as part of their cafeteria plans (also discussed in chapter 2) will be forced to make changes as a result of recent revisions in the tax code. The new provisions reflect the desire of the federal government to limit the spread of most existing plans out of the concern that they result in revenue losses to the federal treasury and also stimulate medical expenses. Whether or not they are inflationary is hotly debated. Nonetheless, in order for employees to be eligible for favorable tax treatment, the medical expense account plans will have to be prefunded through payroll deduction, with the employee making the election to participate before the beginning of the plan year. Any money that remains in the account at the end of the year, meaning that it has not been used for medical expenses, will be forfeited. In contrast, under most plans now in existence, the unused portion either accumulates or is paid to the employee. The effect of the change is to make medical expense accounts less desirable to both employers and employees, and it will be interesting to see how many plans continue to operate.

ALTERNATIVE DELIVERY SYSTEMS: HMOs AND PPOs

The major development regarding health maintenance organizations (HMOs) is the upsurge in enrollment, which reached 12.5 million in 1983, a net increase of 1.7 million. This represents a 15.3 percent rise over 1982, the fastest growth rate since 1978 (InterStudy, 1984).

Employer support of HMOs is one reason for these increases, as illustrated by the recent actions of two companies. First, Ford Motor

Company mounted an intensive campaign to promote HMO enrollment. It contracts with a total of 26 HMOs. For 12 of these, employees pay a share of the HMO's premium. Enrollment in these HMOs increased 50 percent during the last open enrollment period. For the remaining 14, the company pays the full premium because the HMO premium is below the company's contribution to its conventional insurance plan. Enrollment in these HMOs increased an astounding 250 percent, and, currently, 20 percent of all Ford employees with access to an HMO have enrolled in one. Second, new employees of Lockheed at three major locations—Burbank and Sunnyvale, California, and Marietta, Georgia—will be offered only HMO options for the first year of employment. After that they will be able to switch to the company's indemnity plan.

Preferred provider organizations (PPOs) in various stages of planning, development, and initial marketing continue to outnumber manyfold those with actual enrollment. We estimate that, at most, 20 or 30 have enrollment in excess of 2,000. At the same time, more are becoming successful; these appear to be geographically concentrated, e.g., in California, Ohio, and Florida. One trend is towards greater involvement of insurance carriers than was true a year ago (e.g., Metropolitan, Prudential, Pacific Mutual, Fireman's Fund, and the Blue Cross plans in California and Virginia).

New variants of the PPO are also evolving. For example, in January 1984, Stouffers entered into a contract with the six PPOs in Cleveland that comprise the Emerald Health Network. Employees enroll in the PPO as an alternative to either the indemnity plan or the HMOs that are offered. Unlike most PPO arrangements, reimbursements are not made to enrollees for services rendered by nonparticipating providers except in cases of emergency and services out of the area. This approach is sometimes referred to as an "exclusive provider option." As another example, two Taft-Hartley trust funds in Sacramento, California, are in the process of negotiating contracts with individual hospitals and physicians. They will neither reimburse for care outside of the provider network that they establish nor offer an alternative indemnity plan. This approach is commonly referred to as an "exclusive provider organization."

The growth of data systems and employer interest in utilization review (UR), described below, can be further expected to stimulate the growth of preferred provider arrangements. As profiling becomes more widespread, employers will have the data upon which to base decisions to favor certain providers over others. The availability of this data will naturally lead to instituting plan design incentives and disincentives that do so, with some employers working through organized provider groups and others dealing directly with individual providers or with a network of providers formed by carriers, third party administrators, or other nonprovider organizations.

One question is the likely impact of PPOs on HMOs. One PPO reports that, among the groups with which it has contracts, the growth in HMO enrollment has been stemmed because employees with the PPO option who use participating providers have coverage that is as comprehensive as that offered by HMOs and, in addition, have access to nonparticipating providers if they are willing to pay cost sharing. On the other hand, the widespread attention that PPOs have attracted has heightened employers' awareness of alternative delivery systems generally. Because of their skepticism of PPOs, particularly the fact that the PPO does not absorb risk, many employers have, instead, favored HMOs.

The future of the PPO nationally is itself uncertain. Some believe that the PPO will become a major financing and delivery mechanism in its own right that will rival the HMO in terms of numbers of patients seen. Others contend that the PPO concept will succeed only in isolated circumstances and will not be a major force. Still others argue that most successful PPOs will evolve into HMOs.

Our own view is that PPOs are a precursor to a more complex world and will succeed in some locations but not others. More importantly, many are likely to evolve a broad set of "product lines," which could include, in addition to the conventional PPO structure, an HMO, an exclusive provider organization, and various forms of risk sharing with purchasers of care. The common theme of these product lines is that they all combine financing with delivery.

UTILIZATION REVIEW

The 1983–1985 period has two major foci of activity for utilization review: (1) implementation of the federal professional review organization (PRO) program and (2) the maturation of data systems for utilization monitoring and management.

As this book goes to press, many professional standards review organizations (PSROs) are competing to become designated as the new PROs. Ironically, their competition is, in many instances, the same medical societies that historically opposed both the original PSRO program and its most recent incarnation (in 1982) as PRO. Medical societies generally have accepted the inevitability of some form of government review and are cognizant of the increasing private sector demands for UR. From the perspective of employers who have supported the UR movement, the most interesting aspect of this conflict between PSROs and medical societies is the fact that both groups are seeking, rather than avoiding, employers who want to participate in review.

While the political battles over PRO designation and data access have been increasing, computerized systems for utilization and cost data manipulation have become much more sophisticated. The implications for UR are significant. One trend is toward greater simplicity. There are now several firms that base their UR system on telephone monitoring and approvals: the patient or the provider is responsible for telephoning a central 800-number for authorization to enter the hospital. In some cases, this telephone call generates all future UR activity. This approach has the obvious advantages of offering nationwide coverage through a central staff, the standardization of protocols, and a service that is less expensive than one which requires on-site professional review teams. (Examples of companies that have implemented, or are now implementing, such a program include General Mills, Armco Steel, Stouffers, and RCA.) Computerized data systems that generate provider profiles and permit easy comparison of treatment plans with area, regional, and national norms have been essential for the growth of the 800-number approach.

While some have been attracted to the simplicity and relative low cost of the telephone predetermination systems, others have focused on either concurrent review or retrospective analysis. Again, new data systems are critical. UR is advancing from an era of minimal sophistication in which reviewers had little more upon which to rely than their own experience and powers of persuasion. Today, a review group can use data systems for area population-based utilization analysis, hospital-specific cost and treatment profiles (e.g., Health Systems International), and claims analysis by DRG that can include the complete performance record of every physician (e.g., Health Data Institute, MedStat, Co-Med).

Controlled studies have not been performed that show an employer either what data system to buy or which UR method will produce the best results. Data systems are maturing faster than any study could reflect and, fortunately, all of the UR methods show considerable payoff for the purchaser. Four trends are noteworthy. First, integrated UR systems are becoming more prevalent. Precertification programs will become widespread for a growing list of procedures. These programs will be integrated into the design of the benefit packages, which have cost sharing penalties if the prescribed precertification procedures are not followed. Concurrent review will be targeted to those facilities, physicians, and diagnoses where the data reveal patterns of excess. Retrospective analysis will also serve to generate provider profiles and identify questionable patterns of care. On its own, retrospective analysis has been demonstrated by groups, such as the Delaware Review Organization, a PSRO, to reduce hospital use by placing aberrant physicians on notice.

Second, given the increasing pressures on physicians from the combined forces of regulation and competition, UR will, we predict, become a cost-management mechanism mutually supported by physicians as well as purchasers. In Texas, the cooperative precertification program of LTV and the Texas Medical Foundation is an example. The program is called "Advanced Approval for Medical Benefits" and covers extended care, home health care, hospices, mental health, surgery, and substance abuse treatment in addition to hospital inpatient care. If procedures that can be performed safely on an outpatient basis are performed in the hospital, all reimbursement for room and board charges are denied. Since August 1983, LTV has experienced a reduction of admissions per 1,000 employees from 450 to 190, and cost per admission has been reduced over 30 percent.

Third, UR will be an increasingly powerful tool, again due to better data, for reducing medically unjustified variations in practice patterns. For example, the variation in outpatient surgery rates by county has been analyzed for Utah by the statewide coalition there. The following illustrates some of the findings for two pairs of counties:

Procedure	Salt Lake/Davis	Weber/N. Davis
Tonsillectomy & adenoidectomy	68.0%	7.4%
Fallopian tube transection	66.0	96.0

Results also show one hospital performing 83 percent of tonsillectomies and adenoidectomies on an outpatient basis, and another hospital performing less than 20 percent (Utah Health Cost Management Foundation 1982).

Physician behavior can also be altered by disseminating research findings on medical practice outcomes. Again in Utah, less than 8 percent of inguinal hernia repairs are performed on an outpatient basis, despite more than 25 years of reported experience supporting the efficacy of this procedure (Lichtenstein 1984). A Salt Lake City physician recently duplicated those results, and Utah employers are being shown that a longstanding style of practice that reflects the norm may generate unnecessary costs. As another example, physicians at Duke University, according to studies performed by Gaylen Wagner, M.D., are discharging uncomplicated heart attack cases within 5 days of admission rather than the standard 12–14 days, with equivalent or improved outcomes (Wagner 1984).

Finally, UR will become increasingly common for disciplines, such as mental health and substance abuse treatment, that have traditionally been poorly reviewed. Paul Gertman's work at Health Data Institute has recently shown that employees with alcoholism treatment claims consumed an average of 11 times more medical care than those who had no such claims (Rosenbloom and Gertman 1984). Benefits may need to be redesigned to restructure the coverage of mental health services before the results of UR analysis can have its full impact.

As always, the long-run success of UR in constraining communitywide costs will depend in large measure on the availability of efficient alternative delivery settings, reimbursement that provides incentives for using those alternatives, and a process for shrinking the increasingly excessive acute care hospital capacity.

COALITIONS

Over the past year, the coalition movement surprised its critics: the rate of growth in numbers, sophistication, and aggressiveness increased. Many observers had suggested that the stronger economy combined with reductions in the rate of medical care cost escalation would cause employer interest in coalitions to wane.

Instead, the opposite occurred. Improved economic conditions both provided more resources for coalition activities and made the gap between inflation in the economy as a whole and medical care cost escalation all the more apparent. Cost-management successes have had the effect of showing purchasers that their efforts were worthwhile. Media coverage and conference speakers across the nation began to replace stories about the potential of coalitions with examples of specific achievements. In turn, this has led communities without coalitions to feel behind the times. By the end of 1984, coalitions will be functioning in roughly 200 communities, and intrastate networks are growing in popularity as states such as North Carolina find themselves with more than 20 separate groups.

The movement is having an impact at the state level as governors become increasingly aware of medical care cost pressures. No longer is a governor likely to call in the medical industry for private meetings or create a task force with token business involvement. The new governor's task force in Missouri, appointed by Governor Christopher Bond, is a good example. This group is cochaired by business leaders. Task force members include staff and employer representatives from the major coalitions in St. Louis and Kansas City as well as organized labor. The membership is approximately two-thirds purchaser and one-third provider. Further, the representatives of the St. Louis Medical Society and the Missouri Hospital Association view their role as leaders for the future rather than defenders of the past. A central point of this development is that the coalitions need help from the state, and the state knows that it cannot achieve comprehensive reform without the coalitions.

Evidence of the new power of the combination of public and private purchasers has not been lost on state legislatures. A year ago, the role of the business community in obtaining passage of an all-payer law in Massachusetts and a full disclosure law in Iowa were the leading examples of coalition influence at the state level. Today, coalitions in South Florida and Connecticut have achieved legislative victories; the coalition in Arizona assumed a leadership role in obtaining the required number of signatures to force legislative action on an all-payer system of hospital reimbursement; and coalitions are deeply involved in all-payer legislative battles in Illinois and Pennsylvania, among other states.

Another significant development has been the evolution of coalition leaders. Coalitions began with the impetus of a few employers and even fewer national health policy personalities. In 1984, coalition staff leaders are emerging as a new force. Top staffers in Iowa, Utah, New York, Lehigh Valley, St. Louis, San Diego, Portland (Oregon), Seattle, Minneapolis, Hartford, South Florida, and Massachusetts now constitute a new cadre of health policy and cost-management experts whose experience is more diverse than that of any single interest group.

In the early 1990s the coalition movement will have entered its second decade. By then, today's trends will have emerged as norms, and the movement will be seen as a mature force in medical economics and health policy. Between now and then a number of exciting developments are likely.

Virtually every major metropolitan area and many smaller communities will have a group devoted to medical care cost management. In addition, states will typically have numerous city and county groups in a network related to a statewide purchaser group that, in turn, works with a statewide multiparty coalition including the legislature and the governor's office. Also, regional coordinating groups, similar to the Midwest Business Group on Health, will cover the country. Finally, at the national level, the policy exchange program of the Washington Business Group on Health will have evolved into a policy network that provides coalitions with an opportunity to express their views on all relevant government regulations and legislation at every stage of their development.

Currently, participation of unions in coalitions is spotty. However, their sophistication and level of participation will increase as they unite with employers to address cost-management issues out of concern for the proportion of take-home pay that health benefits and out-of-pocket health care costs represent.

Evaluations of cost-management strategies, now in their infancy, will guide coalition agendas. These evaluations will be aided by nationwide systems for sharing computerized data necessary for price, service, utilization, and quality comparisons among providers.

High on the agendas will be reform and improved management of the disability and workers' compensation programs. Also, more of the focus of cost management will have shifted from the hospital to the outpatient setting, which in many ways is more complex and fragmented. This will entail new approaches to utilization review, diagnostic reporting, claims management, precertification, facilities' cost-effectiveness measurement, and patient care norms.

Finally, increased attention will be paid to worker productivity issues, worksite health hazards, and the role of business in public health issues, such as family violence and infant mortality. The most innovative groups will have begun to relate changes in the medical care system with reform of public education, transportation, housing, and employment.

Employers are the reasons coalitions exist, regardless of their structure. With the economic power that coalitions represent comes a great responsibility. Coalitions can be a force for good by enhancing quality of care, excising waste, improving the balance between competition and regulation, and preserving the ethical commitment to those who must depend on public support for access to care. However, any group with that much power will surely find itself held accountable for any abuse of power. The more successful cost-management strategies become, the more effort those involved must make to be guided, not just by their short-term bottom line, but also by a long-term partnership with their employees, retirees, dependents, and fellow citizens united in a common cause: the pursuit of a healthy population served by a medical industry that responds to the incentives of an efficient marketplace and responsible regulation.

WORKSITE WELLNESS

A review of trends in worksite wellness over the past year shows that the movement is expanding in that there are more programs in more companies, the business of health promotion is flourishing, degree programs are entering the academic mainstream, and the evidence of the economic payoff for prevention is becoming more compelling. In addition, the more sophisticated programs are gaining greater focus, risk assessment is increasingly viewed as essential, and the professionalism of worksite managers is increasing with a simultaneous narrowing of their responsibilities to "only" wellness. What had been an add-on of uncertain value is increasingly regarded as a basic component of normal health benefits.

Additional trends that have gained currency during that past year include the broadening of prevention programs to include older workers, giving priority to those identified as being at high risk of cancer or cardiovascular disease, using medical care cost-management data to target wellness programs, and recognizing the impact of corporate culture on health and productivity. These four threads represent a shifting of the leading programs away from being focused on recreation or fitness and limited to headquarters employees. Increasingly, programs are viewed as appropriate for the whole workforce as well as valuable for families and retirees.

Evaluation of programs is gaining favor, although the cost of timely comprehensive longitudinal studies remains prohibitive for most employers. The new Washington Business Group on Health journal, *Corporate Commentary*, the first issue of which appeared in June 1984, is devoted to wellness program evaluations and evaluation methodology. The rapid growth of the publication's circulation is one indicator of the appetite for evidence of program effectiveness.

Corporate culture is the topic which, to many, still seems more like a fad than solid benefits programming. However, it has captured the attention of leading health and business experts and is increasingly the subject of media scrutiny. Whether it is Ford's use of quality circles to help improve worksite safety and reduce conditions that the employees perceive as unsafe or Tenneco's enthusiastic effort to make fitness a regular part of the workday, more and more companies accept that there is a strong link between the quality of work, the quality of the workplace, and worker health.

Perhaps the most impressive culture-oriented program was developed by Marc Michaelson for General Dynamics in San Diego. It entails an integrated approach to total human performance and involves everything from spirituality to physical fitness, financial fitness to sense of job worth, and family fitness to personal creativity. Employees run many of the programs, provide much of the financing, and are encouraged to create program refinements.

Worksite wellness is becoming less a curiosity and more the norm. Unions are increasingly receptive, screening technology is improving, examples of success are more frequent and accessible, and the public demand for a healthy workplace is louder than ever. Corporate chairmen are more willing to speak publicly about prevention, and the health insurance industry is on the verge of offering meaningful incentives for healthy life styles. Together these advances suggest a strong future for worksite wellness. But, like the rest of the medical industry, as wellness moves into the mainstream, it, too, will be subject to greater competition and demands for accountability.

CONCLUSION

Increasingly, firms are not only developing comprehensive strategies for managing their health benefits but are also integrating those efforts with the management of disability-related costs, such as those associated with both short- and long-term sick leave and workers' compensation expenses. In addressing disability programs, they are emulating the emerging experiences of UR and other aspects of health benefits management. For example, they are developing protocols for the number of sick-leave days that are appropriate for a given condition. They are profiling employees to identify those with aberrant absence patterns (e.g., sick leave that occurs primarily on Fridays and Mondays) and doctors who appear overly lenient in certifying disability. Some companies have appointed a panel of doctors to certify, independent of the employee's personal physician, the need for sick leave or medical care. For example, Chrysler and the United Automobile Workers have agreed to such a panel, and they jointly participate in the process of selecting physicians to serve on it. Importantly, the data and experience from these programs are a critical element in the feedback loop to structure worksite wellness and occupational safety programs.

Large companies are increasingly encountering two dilemmas in managing their health benefits. The first, mentioned in chapter 9, is whether individual units of a company, such as particular plants or divisions, should be held accountable for health care expenditures by attributing to them the actual claims experience of their employees, even if they do not control the benefit package or select the organization that does claims processing. Although the health benefits staffs of most large corporations are far more sophisticated than was the case a few years ago, that sophistication is often limited to the headquarters of the corporation or, at best, to its major subsidiaries. At the same time, a large share of ongoing management decisions that affect spending occurs at the local level, including how to structure employee information campaigns that are provider-specific; which providers to favor through preferred provider arrangements; how aggressive to be in conducting UR; whether to participate actively in health care coalitions; whether to sit on hospital or health planning boards; and whether to engage in local battles regarding health facilities planning, capacity reduction, hospital rate setting, and insurance laws. Alcoa and DuPont are two companies that have recently switched responsibility for health benefit expenses to holding units below the corporate level.

The second is whether firms should maintain nationally uniform benefit programs. Many corporations (or their individual subsidiaries) have adhered to the position that any benefit must be available to all employees, and, as a corollary, no differentiation should exist among employees in terms of the manner in which they are affected by cost-containment or benefit-enhancement measures. At the same time, comprehensive health benefits managers must be cognizant of local circumstances. Some measures may be economically justified only in areas of high employment concentration, such as certain elements of a wellness program. Opportunities to alter plan design to achieve savings through contracts with preferred provider organizations will not arise in all communities. The need for, and appropriate structure of, an effective UR program will differ among communities. As a final example, the feasibility of having on-site medical care will also differ. Many corporations are now wrestling with the tradeoffs between the desirability from an employee relations perspective of maintaining complete uniformity and the concomitant loss of cost-management opportunities that uniformity may entail.

REFERENCES

Corporate Commentary 1(June 1984).
Lichtenstein, I. Presented at Pew Fellowship Seminar, May 24–25, 1984, Boston.
National HMO Census—1983. Excelsior, Minn.: InterStudy, 1984.
Rosenbloom, D.L., and P.M. Gertman. "Pinpointing High Users of Health Care." *Business and Health* 1(July/August 1984): 17–21.
Utah Health Cost Management Foundation, unpublished findings, 1982.
Wagner, G. Presented at Pew Fellowship Seminar, May 24–25, 1984, Boston.

Index

About the Authors

PETER D. FOX is a vice-president of Lewin and Associates, a Washington-based research and consulting firm, where he has performed work for a variety of public and private clients, including the U.S. Department of Health and Human Services, several large health care manufacturers and distributors, hospitals, a long-term care facility, health care coalitions, the National Association of Private Psychiatric Hospitals, the Pharmaceutical Manufacturers Association, the United Mine Workers Funds, the Hartford Foundation, the city of New York, and the state of Alaska. For 11 years prior to joining the firm in 1981, he served in a variety of positions in the federal government, most recently as director of the Office of Policy Analysis in the Health Care Financing Administration. He has also worked for Stanford Research Institute (now called SRI International) and the Stanford University School of Medicine. Dr. Fox has published articles on such topics as alternative delivery systems, physician reimbursement, physician utilization patterns, mental health program evaluation, and long-term care. He has a Ph.D. in business administration from Stanford University, an M.S. in management from MIT, and an A.B. from Haverford College.

WILLIS B. GOLDBECK is the president of the Washington Business Group on Health, the national health policy organization for major employers, which he started in 1974. Previously, he served as special assistant for research and technology at the U.S. Department of Housing and Urban Development, was a correspondent for *Time Magazine*, and was executive vice-president of the Center for Responsive Technology. Mr. Goldbeck has also served on the Board of Directors of the American Health Planning Association, the Washington Hospital Center, and the National Rehabilitation Hospital. He has been the vice-chairman of the Policy Advisory Committee of the Joint Commission on Accreditation of Hospitals and is on the faculty of Boston University's School of Public Health.

JACOB J. SPIES is currently President of Co-Med, Inc., a health care management and development firm headquartered in Columbus, Ohio. At the time this book was written, he was deputy director of Boston University's Center for Industry and Health Care and was responsible for the center's corporate consulting activities. Clients have included IBM, Deere, Gillette, AT&T, International Harvester, DuPont, Armco, Alcoa, Mobil Oil, General Electric, New York Telephone, and Citibank. He has served on various government commissions, including the Wisconsin Hospital Rate Review Commission and the Massachusetts Group Insurance Commission as well as on governor's task forces on health care costs in Wisconsin, Florida, and Vermont. He has published numerous articles on corporate cost containment and HMO development. Mr. Spies holds a B.S. degree in corporate management-insurance from the University of Wisconsin School of Commerce and is adjunct assistant professor at the Boston University Schools of Medicine and Public Health.